More praise for

Tell Me What You Want

"Have a deep, dark sex fantasy that you've never shared with anyone? Turns out, you're not alone. Most people are afraid their sex
fantasies are abnormal, but Justin Lehmiller's newest book reveals
that understanding your erotic imaginings, and sharing them with
your sex partner, might be the best, healthiest thing you do all
year. *Tell Me What You Want* educates, titillates, thrills, and guides
us down a marvelous, sexy path that ends in acceptance of those
naughty secrets in the basements of our minds."

—David J. Ley, PhD, author of
The Myth of Sex Addiction

"Lehmiller's smart, warm, sex-positive book breaks the toxic si-
lence around our sexual fantasies. Reading it may be the best
thing you ever do for your sex life, your relationships, and your
self-acceptance."

—Geoffrey Miller, author of *The
Mating Mind, Spent,* and *Mate*

"Lehmiller's groundbreaking book points to an alarmin
tween the conversations we're having about sex and th
tion we should be having about sex. It provides the nud
to change the conversation—and, in doing so, to live he
ter lives."

—Eli J. Finkel, F
Psychology, Northwestern

"As Justin Lehmiller, PhD, explains so insightfully in his fascinating new book, *Tell Me What You Want*, most of us have lots of turn-ons that would definitely not earn the *Good Housekeeping* seal of approval."

—Ari Tuckman's *Psychology Today* blog, "Sex Matters"

"Lehmiller uses his book as a vehicle to explain how common some sexual fantasies are—not to mention fantasizing in general—and to help the reader better fulfill their own desires....Lehmiller's calm and logical approach to understanding sexuality and improving sexual satisfaction...is exemplified on nearly every page."

—Of Sex and Love blog

"Attempts to dispel stereotypes, shed light on why so many of us imagine similar scenarios, and serve as a guide to helping us talk about what we desire."

—*Boston Globe*

"If you've ever had a sexual fantasy and thought, 'Oh God, what's wrong with me?' a quick read of *Tell Me What You Want*...might ease your mind....Lehmiller isn't just putting out a compendium of our raciest thoughts; he tries to explain what those thoughts do for the health of our psyches....He gives concrete advice."

—*New York Times Book Review*

"A book that will be reassuring for therapists and patients alike....Lively....Valuable and enjoyable. The writing is clear, informal, and describes human sexuality in a recognizable fashion."

—*The Therapist*

ALSO BY JUSTIN J. LEHMILLER

The Psychology of Human Sexuality

Tell Me What You Want

THE SCIENCE OF SEXUAL DESIRE AND HOW IT
CAN HELP YOU IMPROVE YOUR SEX LIFE

by Justin J. Lehmiller, PhD

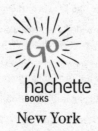

hachette
BOOKS

New York

We are the recorders and reporters of facts, not the judges of the behaviors we describe.

—Alfred Kinsey

Hachette Go, an imprint of Hachette Books
Hachette Book Group
1290 Avenue of the Americas, New York, NY 10104
HachetteGo.com
Facebook.com/HachetteGo
Instagram.com/HachetteGo

Printed in the United States of America
First Trade Paperback Edition: July 2020

Published by Hachette Go, an imprint of Perseus Books, LLC, a subsidiary of Hachette Book Group, Inc. The Hachette Go name and logo is a trademark of the Hachette Book Group.

The Hachette Speakers Bureau provides a wide range of authors for speaking events. To find out more, go to www.hachettespeakersbureau.com or call (866) 376-6591.

The publisher is not responsible for websites (or their content) that are not owned by the publisher.

Library of Congress Cataloging-in-Publication Data has been applied for.

ISBNs: 978-0-7382-3495-3 (hardcover), 978-0-7382-3496-0 (paperback), 978-0-7382-3497-7 (ebook)
LSC-C
10 9 8 7 6 5 4 3 2 1

Contents

Preface

Fantasy, Fear, and Freud

"I'm scared people will find out what I masturbate to."

So said actor Donald Glover in an emotionally raw Instagram post.[1] With a simple photograph of a handwritten note, Glover perfectly distilled the profound sense of dread so many of us feel about our own sexual desires. Instead of seeing them as something to be shared or possibly even acted upon, we tend to tuck them away in the deepest recesses of our minds because we view them as nothing more than a source of potential shame and embarrassment.

Social scientists have long known that sexual fantasies go hand in hand with feelings of guilt and anxiety, having published dozens of academic journal articles over the years supporting this conclusion.[2] Anecdotally, I have also observed this among readers of my website, Sex and Psychology—a site I created to provide science-based sex ed for adults. Shortly after posting my first article, I began to receive emails from people all over the world who were worried about their own fantasies or, sometimes, the fantasies of their partners. Women whose most arousing fantasies involve themes of rape, heterosexual men who get off on transsexual porn, married women who have discovered that their husbands enjoy cross-dressing, and men who want to share their wives and girlfriends with other men—they all want to know where these fantasies came from and, more often than not, what's wrong with them.

Their concern is hardly surprising. For centuries, political, religious, and medical authorities in the United States have argued that what's acceptable to desire when it comes to sex is very narrow. They've pretty much told us that we shouldn't do anything other than put penises in vaginas and even that, ideally, should only take place within the confines of a heterosexual, monogamous marriage. Desires for any other sexual activities have been deemed unnatural, immoral, and unhealthy—and we've been discouraged from acting on them with threats of criminal prosecution and divine retribution.

There are obviously many sources of blame in America's legacy of sex shame, but I want to focus on one here that has a tendency to get overlooked: our mental health community. Psychologists and psychiatrists have contributed in a major way to the stigmatization of many perfectly normal sexual desires. They have done so by advancing the notion that our sexual fantasies are a source of danger. This can be traced back to Sigmund Freud, who famously wrote more than a century ago that "a happy person never fantasizes, only a dissatisfied one."[3] Freud believed fantasies were a window into our psychological health and that they were necessarily revealing of deeper troubles. According to his view, someone who has a lot of self-loathing, for instance, might develop fantasies about being used, humiliated, or punished.

Well, as you may know, Freud had a lot to say about sex—but much of it was just plain wrong. For example, he argued that the "mature" woman reaches orgasm through vaginal penetration, not clitoral stimulation. He also argued that male homosexuality results from growing up with a domineering mother and an absentee father. There was never much scientific evidence to support these claims, and the same is true of his views on sexual fantasy.

Although the American mental health community has increasingly moved away from most of Freud's claims, it continues to instill a sense of fear and shame about sexual fantasy to this day by formally declaring numerous sexual desires to be unusual, or, in the psychological lexicon, *paraphilic*. According to the *Diagnostic and Statistical Manual of Mental Disorders* (DSM), the bible that American psychologists and psychiatrists live by, a paraphilia is a preference for any kind of nonnormative sexual activity or target. The current version of the DSM mentions eight specific paraphilias, including *sadism* and *masochism*, which refer to sexual gratification achieved through giving and receiving pain, respectively; *transvestism*, which refers to obtaining sexual arousal through cross-dressing; and *fetishism*, which refers to sexual desire for a nonsexual object or body part.

The DSM is just the tip of the iceberg when it comes to the number of sexual desires the mental health community has deemed unusual, though. For example, the technical handbook *Forensic and Medico-legal Aspects of Sexual Crimes and Unusual Sexual Practices*, by Dr. Anil Aggrawal, details a whopping 547 distinct paraphilias! Many of the entries on Aggrawal's list would seemingly live up his book's title, such as *vomerophilia*, which refers to being sexually aroused by vomit; *eproctophilia*, an intense sexual attraction to flatulence; and *zoonecrophilia*, the desire to have sex with dead animals. Others, however, don't sound out of the ordinary at all, such as *coprolalia*, which refers to sexual arousal derived from the use of obscene language; *sitophilia*, which refers to arousal from the use of food during sexual activity; and *neo-philia*, which refers to sexual arousal stemming from novelty or change. Wait—what? If we take this list at face values, it implies that anyone who is really into dirty talk, who loves using whipped cream or other edibles during foreplay, or who finds sexual routines to be dull is, well, kind of a pervert. Really?

The truth is that many of the entries on Aggrawal's list—which also includes (gasp!) desires for oral and anal sex—are actually very commonly desired and practiced behaviors. Some of the paraphilias listed in the DSM are, too, such as the desire to mix pleasure and pain. Case in point: perhaps you've heard of the phenomenally popular book—and film—*Fifty Shades of Grey*? In other words, a lot of sexual desires have been deemed unusual despite being anything but. This raises an important question: What is "normal" when it comes to sex, and who gets to decide that?

Psychologists and psychiatrists have been telling us what's normal and what isn't for a very long time. Unfortunately, they haven't necessarily approached this matter objectively. Basically, whenever they've encountered something that doesn't *appear* normal to them, they have erred on the side of calling it a paraphilia, even in the absence of evidence that a given desire is rare or unusual. This freewheeling, arbitrary tendency to label desire after desire as paraphilic has had the problematic effect of stigmatizing far too many sexual interests because, for almost the entire time the DSM has been in existence, the term *paraphilia* has been synonymous with *mental disorder.*

Look no further than the 1950s and '60s, when homosexuality was classified as a paraphilia in the DSM. This led the public to view being gay as a disorder. As long as homosexuality was considered a mental illness, what need was there for society to address gay rights? It's not far off to say that, at that time, granting workplace protections and marriage equality to gays would have been seen as tantamount to indulging the delusions of paranoid schizophrenics through legislative action. The DSM provided cover for America to dismiss gays' pursuit of equal rights and to instead argue that the only thing they really needed was therapy to "correct" their sexual orientation. In other words, it allowed the country as a whole to say, "The gays are the ones who need to change, not us." Taking homosexuality out of the DSM was therefore a truly significant event. With the "disorder" title stripped away, people had no choice but to start taking the concerns of gays and lesbians seriously. For this reason, the declassification of homosexuality as a mental illness (which formally occurred in 1973) was arguably the most significant milestone in the American gay rights movement.

The sexual desires that appeared alongside homosexuality in earlier versions of the DSM and that are still considered paraphilias today—things like foot fetishes, cross-dressing, sadism, and masochism—continue to be regarded by much of American society as perversions or mental illnesses. The same goes for the hundreds upon hundreds of other, less notorious desires that others have declared paraphilic. This widespread stigmatization of sexual desire perpetuated by the mental health community is not only arbitrary and unscientific—it is actively harmful to Americans' sex lives and relationships. The more shame, embarrassment, and anxiety people feel about their sexual desires, the more likely they are to avoid talking about sex at all and to experience sexual performance difficulties, finding it challenging to become (or stay) aroused or to reach orgasm. Poor communication coupled with sexual performance issues can, in turn, snowball into major relationship problems and, in severe cases, even precipitate a breakup or divorce.

Psychology should be helping, not hurting, people's sex lives and relationships. The field has certainly done a lot to help over the years—don't get me wrong about that. But when it comes to how psychology has treated sexual desire and fantasy, there is still much that could stand to change. In particular, we need to fundamentally reevaluate what a "normal" sexual desire is and be far more cautious when it comes to throwing that paraphilia label around.

In order to do this, we must begin by coming to a better understanding of the nature of sexual desire. Which desires are common and which ones are truly rare? And how much does the prevalence of a given desire matter, anyway, when it comes to how we evaluate it? Just because a desire is rare, does that mean it's necessarily unhealthy or inappropriate to act upon? Also, how do sexual desires differ for men and women? What about for persons of different ages and sexual orientations? Why do different people want different things in the first place? And is it a good idea to share and act on your sexual fantasies? If so, how the heck do you go about doing that in a safe way?

There are currently far too many gaps in the scientific literature for us to answer these questions, which is why I spent more than a year conducting the largest and most comprehensive survey of Americans' sexual fantasies ever undertaken. The results of this survey will help to fill some of the holes in our knowledge. Not only will this give us a better understanding of what Americans really want when it comes to sex, including what's normal and what isn't, but—even better—we can potentially use this information to improve our sex lives and relationships.

Introduction

The Largest Survey of Sexual Fantasies in America

In the pages that follow, I will offer an analysis of the largest-ever survey of Americans' sexual fantasies, which will show how psychology, evolution, and culture shape not just what we fantasize about but who we want to be with and how we see ourselves. I have identified seven major themes that characterize the nature of sexual desire in America today, each of which I'll explore in detail, carefully describing their primary features (with details drawn from the actual fantasy narratives submitted by survey participants) and their underlying psychology. I'll use my survey results to help you better understand why some things are a turn-on to some but a turn-off to others.

This book is built around a massive survey of more than 350 questions taken by more than four thousand Americans, including persons from all fifty states. Although the sample is not necessarily representative of the US population, it does consist of an incredibly diverse group of individuals. Participants ranged in age from eighteen to eighty-seven and had occupations spanning everything from cashiers at McDonald's to homemakers to physicians to lawyers. The group included all sexual and gender identities, political and religious affiliations, and relationship types, from singles to swingers.

This study is unique not just for the size and diversity of the sample but also for the scope of the survey itself and what it can tell us. In addition to being queried in great detail about their biggest sexual fantasy of all time, participants were asked how frequently they fantasize about hundreds of different people, places, and things. Included in this were a wide range of sexual acts and settings, body parts and objects, as well as specific persons, from porn stars to celebrities to politicians. In addition, participants were asked to carefully describe what the typical men and women in their fantasies look like, from their height, weight, race, and hair color to the presence or absence of pubic hair to the size of their breasts and genitals. Detailed sexual histories, psychological profiles, and demographic characteristics were also collected. All in all, this survey offers an unprecedented look into our fantasy worlds and what they reveal about us. Below are just a few of the many key insights:

- Almost all Americans who took this survey (97 percent) reported having sexual fantasies—and most reported having them frequently. The vast majority said they fantasize somewhere between several times per week and several times per day. To fantasize—and to fantasize often—is therefore to be human.

- Sex with multiple partners is a staple of Americans' fantasies. When asked to describe their favorite sexual fantasy of all time, group sex was by far the most common theme to emerge. In addition, when asked whether they had *ever* fantasized about different forms of group sex, 89 percent reported fantasizing about threesomes, 74 percent about orgies, and 61 percent about gangbangs. Although men were more likely to have all of these multipartner fantasies than women, it will surprise many to learn that the majority of women reported having each of these sex fantasies as well.

- Sadomasochism, or the desire to link pleasure and pain during sex, is another extremely popular American fantasy. In fact, 60 percent of participants reported having fantasized about inflicting physical pain on someone else during sex, while 65 percent reported having fantasized about receiving physical pain during sex. Believe it or not, women were more likely than men to have fantasized about both giving and receiving pain, though the gender difference was larger for the latter. With numbers like these, it should come as no surprise that *Fifty Shades of Grey* had such cultural resonance.

- Hollywood might give you the impression that Americans are fantasizing about celebrities more than anyone else, but that could not be further from the truth. Just 7 percent of participants said that they fantasize about celebrities often, whereas 51 percent said that they fantasize about their current partner often. That's right—we fantasize about real-life, everyday people far more frequently than we fantasize about the Zac Efrons and Scarlett Johanssons of the world. This suggests that our fantasies may be more grounded in reality than you think, at least with respect to whom we want to be with.

- Our porn-viewing habits influence who and what we fantasize about. In fact, one in seven participants said that their biggest sexual fantasy of all time directly stems from something they saw in porn. Pornography consumption is related to the size and shape of the bodies and genitals that appear in our fantasies, too. For instance, the more porn that heterosexual men watch, the bigger women's breasts are in their fantasies. Likewise, the more porn that heterosexual women watch, the bigger men's penises are in their fantasies.

- We often become different people in our sexual fantasies. Most of my participants reported that, when they appear in their own fantasies, they change themselves in some way, whether it's having a different body shape, genital appearance, or personality. As you will see shortly, this tendency to fantasize about changing one's physical or psychological characteristics sometimes reflects deep-seated insecurities.

- Americans' political leanings speak volumes about the nature of their sexual fantasies. For example, compared to Democrats, Republicans were more likely to fantasize about sexual activities that are typically considered immoral—like infidelity and orgies—or taboo—like voyeurism. My research suggests that the more political and moral restrictions we have placed on our sexuality, the more intensely we fantasize about breaking free of them.

- Less than one-third of participants said they had previously acted out their biggest sexual fantasy. The

remainder reported holding back for a range of reasons, but especially due to uncertainty about how to
act on it and fears that one's partner would disapprove
of and/or be unwilling to participate in the activity.

The bulk of this book focuses on participants' biggest sexual fantasies of all time. Believe it or not, one in five women
and one in ten men said that just *thinking* about their biggest
fantasy has brought them to orgasm before, independent of any
genital stimulation. Talk about a major turn-on! But it's not just
that—these fantasies represent most people's plans and yearn-
ings for their future sex lives. More than three-quarters of the
men and women I surveyed hope to eventually act on their favorite sexual fantasies. If we want to understand what Americans truly desire, their biggest fantasies therefore provide an
excellent vantage point. As we explore them in detail, I will ask
questions such as: What is the psychology behind this fantasy?
If you have this fantasy, what does that say about your personality and sexual history? Are we evolutionarily programmed for
this desire?

The book will also look at what happens when people share
their fantasies with others and, further, what happens when
people go as far as to act upon their deepest desires. In many
cases, this can be beneficial for you, your partner, and your relationship. To that end, I will offer practical considerations for
those who want to share their fantasies, as well as advice for
those who want to act them out in a safe way. Although there
are certainly benefits to be had in sharing and/or acting upon
your fantasies, there are risks involved, too, and I'll be sure
to discuss those. I'll also make it clear which fantasies should

never be acted upon and when someone should consider professional help managing their sexual desires. Finally, I'll take a broader look at what we as individuals and as a society can do to bring our fantasies closer to reality while maximizing personal happiness and public health. Keep in mind that with great sex comes great responsibility—we must balance our pursuit of sexual gratification with concern for the health and well-being of both ourselves and our partners.

How the Science of Sexual Desire Can Improve Your Sex Life and Relationship

My goal in sharing these survey results is not simply to titillate readers with people's deepest—and sometimes darkest—sexual secrets. You may certainly be titillated at times, but my bigger hope is that you will walk away with a greater understanding of the nature of sexual desire and, potentially, use that information to enhance your own sexual and romantic life.

Too many Americans have distorted perceptions about which sexual desires are "normal" and the types of things that "should" turn them on, leading them to censor the vast majority of their urges and wants. This stems from the fact that accurate information about sex and sexual desire is hard to come by in the United States these days, owing in large part to an embarrassingly poor school-based sex-education system. Many students receive no sex education at all, and those who do are often subject to a curriculum riddled with scientific inaccuracies and falsehoods that focuses more on teaching students how to avoid sex than how sex happens. As I write this, just twenty-four states and the District of Columbia mandate sex education, and even fewer require the information given to be medically accurate.[1] That's right—some states require sex education but don't care whether the information provided is even correct!

Obviously, there are numerous problems with these courses, but one of the biggest is that they neglect the issue of sexual desire almost entirely. We are taught only what people are supposed to want, not what people *actually* want when it comes to sex. The end result is that when most Americans start having sex, their knowledge about it, and about which sexual feelings and practices are "normal," tends to be very low. Our reluctance to teach students any sexual communication skills other than "just say no" has also led to an odd state of affairs in which Americans find it more challenging to talk about sex (even with their own spouse or partner) than to actually have it.

This lack of sexual knowledge and communication ability has profound consequences for our health and happiness. For instance, when we approach sex by acting without really talking or communicating first, it's inevitable that lines and boundaries will be crossed from time to time—and this may lead to disagreements over whether a given experience was mutually pleasurable and perhaps whether it was even consensual. A poor understanding of sex can also lead to relationship dissatisfaction and conflict. In addition, a restricted view of what is sexually normal can contribute to a lot of sexual hang-ups and insecurities by leading people to perceive their own sexual interests as being outside the mainstream or deviant. These sexual anxieties can, in turn, play a major role in producing difficulties with sexual desire, arousal, and orgasm. Indeed, sex therapists have found that a lack of knowledge, false beliefs, and a fear that one's sexual desires are abnormal are at the root of many sex problems. Believe it or not, treating such difficulties is often as simple as giving clients permission to act on their desires (assuming they involve consensual sexual activities, of course) and providing them with proper sex education.[2]

And yet, unfortunately, most adults who believe their sexual interests are unusual never seek sex therapy. Instead, they typically repress those desires and try to carry on a "normal" sex life. This tends to become unsatisfying very quickly, leading to a steep drop-off in desire for sex with one's partner. Rather than viewing this problem for what it really is—internalized shame about one's sexuality and a lack of sexual communication—people can readily find doctors who will determine it's a matter of "low sex drive," an issue that needs a medical fix rather than a psychological one. Pharmaceutical companies are chomping at the bit to provide a solution, investing heavily in medications such as Addyi (flibanserin) and hormonal therapies expressly designed to stimulate desire for the sex that people stopped having. Big Pharma isn't alone here—the less regulated world of supplements is trying to cash in on this, too. Unfortunately, all of these pills, patches, and potions fail to address the psychological issues that underlie most sexual problems. The end result is that we wind up taking medications that, at best, might spur us into having mediocre sex more often.

That's messed up—and it's probably why the research so far has shown that most medications do little more to increase sexual desire than sugar pills.[3] This isn't surprising when you consider that the real problem for a lot of us isn't that we lack desire per se; it's that we lack desire for what we've been told we *should* want when it comes to sex. All too often, we incorrectly label things like sexual confusion and anxiety as low libido. For instance, straight women who have highly arousing lesbian fantasies or straight men who fantasize about sex with a male-to-female transsexual might find themselves distraught over their "real" sexual identity. That anxiety can, in turn, interfere with desire for sex with a partner or spouse and the ability to enjoy it. Individuals facing such situations frequently lack the confidence to explore or even talk about their true sexual desires because they do not know the "right" way to go about it or are worried about being rejected. In such cases, it is easier and less embarrassing to simply complain to a partner or doctor about low sex drive than own up to one's true desires. But science tells us that these fantasies—*your* fantasies—are, in all likelihood, perfectly normal and healthy—and once you understand how common your sexual fantasies are, where they come from, and their deeper meaning, you will gain the ability to express your sexual desires to others so that you and your partner (or partners) might ultimately achieve greater sexual fulfillment and develop more emotional intimacy than ever before. To bring back our flagging libidos, then, what we really need to do is stop suppressing our deeper desires. We do not need a pill or even a psychotherapist to do this. We just need permission to share what it is that really turns us on—to tell each other what we want.

Of course, while gaining the confidence to share our desires is important, knowing how to respond appropriately when others share their fantasies with you is just as vital. Many people have approached me over the years, distressed at the discovery of their partners' seemingly unusual sexual fantasies. Many readers of my work have conveyed their concerns in anonymous emails, but I've also been pulled aside at dinner parties and at bars by folks who, upon discovering what I do for a living, consume some liquid courage and ask their questions in person. Why were their partners aroused by the thought of watching them having sex with a stranger, they asked, when they found the same scenario threatening? Or why would anyone think it was hot to dress up like an animal during sex, or get off on fondling or sniffing feet or shoes? To them, the desires their partners had shared were a major turn-off, silly at best, and maybe even disturbing. Many had laughed at or shamed their partners, and more than a few were even contemplating breakup or divorce simply because they did not know how to deal with their partners' "abnormal" urges. With just a little more understanding of the incredible diversity of human sexual desire and why this diversity exists in the first place, though, they might never have experienced any distress at all and, quite possibly, may have come to see their partners' disclosure as a valuable opportunity to strengthen mutual trust and intimacy, not to mention a chance to reinvigorate their sex lives.

Ultimately, all of us stand to benefit from having a better understanding of each other's desires, not just because it can potentially improve our sex lives and relationships but also because the more that we can grow what we as a society think of as "normal" when it comes to sex, the less likely it is that our own sexual desires can be used as weapons against us. One of the many things preventing us from sharing our sexual fantasies in the first place is the fear of what others could potentially do with that information. If we think our own desires are weird—and other people do, too—that gives those who know our secrets the ability to use them as ammunition against us. For instance, they could spread rumors or gossip in an attempt to publicly embarrass us. Even worse, they could do things like engage in blackmail or try to use those desires as grounds for denying parental rights in a child custody case (something that, sadly, happens far more often than you might think).[4] By expanding our understanding of "normal" sexual desires, we can limit the degree to which sharing our sexual wants with our partners makes us vulnerable to harm.

In the end, I hope that the confidence and knowledge you derive from reading this book will help you enhance your sex life and develop and maintain more satisfying relationships and marriages in the future. My goal is to help break down the barriers to discussing sexual fantasies that exist in your own life so that you might allow those fantasies—the ones that are safe, legal, and consensual—to become part of your sexual reality.

1

Tell Me What You Want, What You Really, Really Want

How I Got More Than Four Thousand People to Open Up About Their Deepest Sexual Desires

Anyone who's ever taken an introductory psychology course knows that, in classic Freudian psychology, everyone's personality can be broken down into three parts: the id, ego, and superego. The id is the most primitive element, consisting of our wants, needs, and desires, especially those of a sexual nature. Freud claimed that our libido, or sex drive, is fully housed within the id.

In Freud's own words, the id is "a cauldron full of seething excitations" that exists only to gratify its own needs.[1] It operates under the so-called pleasure principle—the idea that every desire should be immediately satisfied, consequences be damned. The id doesn't always get its way, of course. It is kept in check by the ego (our common sense) and superego (our conscience).

As I've already established, I don't agree with Freud on a lot of things, but I think his theory of personality offers a useful metaphor for how the human mind approaches sex. Almost all of us have sexual desires that we want to act on and that we know could bring us great pleasure but that we suppress once we decide they're probably unrealistic or that it would be immoral to act upon them. The end result? What we do (and who we do) in our sex lives isn't necessarily an accurate reflection of our deeper, underlying wants.

So what exactly are our ids craving? What are those things that turn us on but that we're too afraid to share, let alone act upon? I sought to answer these questions by asking thousands of Americans about their biggest sexual fantasies of all time. The result is a revealing look at the nature of the American id—the sexual desires that we secretly love but have been taught to loathe.

We'll get to the gangbangs, whips and chains, and foot fetishes soon enough, but before we do, I need to establish some crucial points so that you have some context for what's ahead. Let me take a few moments to describe what exactly a sexual fantasy is and how I went about gathering information on Americans' deepest sexual desires.

What Is a Sexual Fantasy?

A sexual fantasy is any mental picture that comes to mind while you're awake that ultimately turns you on. I'm not talking about sex dreams that you might have while sleeping—I'm only talking about those thoughts and mental images over which you have conscious control and that generate sexual arousal. Simply put, a fantasy is a conscious thought that makes you feel all hot and bothered, and maybe gets some blood flowing to your genitals, too.

A fantasy and its corresponding feelings of arousal might last mere seconds; you might see an attractive person in passing, for example, and spontaneously imagine seeing that individual in the nude or engaged in some sexual act. Such fantasies and their effects can be very short-lived, ending as soon as something else, like an incoming phone call or text message, claims your attention. Or, if you're undistracted or able to return to that fantasy at a later time, you might craft a long, elaborate fantasy that lasts several minutes, maybe even hours.

You might return to a given fantasy over and over again; in fact, there are even some folks who think about the same exact thing *every* time they masturbate or have sex, something Freudian psychologists have termed the "central masturbation fantasy." But you can also have one-off fantasies, like what you imagined doing with that sexy bartender who served you drinks last Friday night. Either way, because fantasies occur while we're conscious, we have the ability to call them to mind on command. Maybe you're bored and you want to masturbate. Or perhaps you're tired, so you concentrate on one of your favorite fantasies to stay aroused long enough to fulfill your partner's desire for sex. Sometimes, though, our fantasies emerge spontaneously, including in situations where we don't even want to feel aroused—at work or school, for example, or maybe even in the middle of religious services.

It can be difficult to stop thinking about fantasies at such moments, because one of the most common methods people use for turning off their fantasies is suppressing them—and, unfortunately, psychologists have found that suppression isn't a very effective way to take your mind off of anything, whether it's sexual in nature or not. In fact, suppressing thoughts has the

ironic effect of making us *more* likely to think about them later!
One of the earliest demonstrations of this idea was published
by a former colleague of mine at Harvard, Dan Wegner.[2] In a
1987 study, he asked college students to mention aloud every
thought that came to mind over a five-minute period into a recording device. Half of the participants were told to think about
a white bear during this time, while the other half were told to
suppress thoughts of white bears. Participants then engaged
in a second five-minute stream-of-consciousness recording but
were given the opposite instructions: if they were told to suppress thoughts of a white bear in the first round, they were told
to think about a white bear in the second round, and vice versa.
During both sessions, whenever participants thought about a
white bear, their instructions were to ring a bell.

Wegner found that whenever participants were told to suppress their thoughts, they did indeed think about white bears
less often; however, they still rang the bell more than once per
minute on average! Even more importantly, though, those participants who were told to suppress thoughts of white bears in
the first session showed a rebound effect in the second session
in which they thought about white bears more than anyone else
in the study. In short, we don't appear to be very good at ban-
ishing unwanted thoughts, whether they be about white bears
or, presumably, having sex with white bears. If you weren't already thinking about having sex with white bears, you probably
are now. Sorry about that.

Why is our discussion focused strictly on sexual fantasies and
not on sex dreams? One important reason is that the content of our
sex dreams can be very different from our sexual fantasies, in part
because we have no conscious control over them. For instance,

someone might have a dream about having sex with his or her mother or father but never fantasize about that—even just recalling such a dream during waking hours might very well cause disgust or revulsion rather than sexual arousal. In other words, some sex dreams are better thought of as nightmares. Furthermore, although we often associate sex dreams with nocturnal emissions (especially for teenage boys), they don't necessarily lead to prolonged periods of sexual arousal or orgasm the way our fantasies often do. I will stick to fantasies here due to these differences and the fact that, in general, we don't know all that much about how dreams really work. I hate to break it to you, but that dream interpretation manual sitting on your shelf is mostly BS.

What Turns You On? How I Studied Americans' Sexual Fantasies

What do we know about sexual fantasies? Not as much as you might think. After exhaustively reviewing the published research on this subject, I came to the realization that we know surprisingly little about what people today are actually fantasizing about, how people's fantasies are connected to their personalities and sexual histories, and how many people have shared and acted upon their fantasies before. This prompted me to put together the most comprehensive survey ever on this subject. In preparation, I read a bunch of popular men's and women's magazines and visited quite a few porn sites—all for scientific purposes, of course. I wanted to make sure that I didn't miss out on asking about any major fantasy topics.

I began my survey by having participants tell me—in their own words—what it is that they want, what they really, *really* want. Specifically, I had them write out their favorite sexual fantasy of all time in narrative form and then sum up the main idea of that fantasy in a single word, like *threesome,* or *spanking,* or *lesbian.* Then I asked a lot of follow-up questions about that favorite fantasy: Had they ever shared it with someone else or tried to act on it? (If they had, what was it like?) Where did they think this fantasy came from? How did it make them feel?

From there, I tried to learn as much about the people who were taking the survey as I could, asking questions about their age, gender, race, sexual orientation, educational background, political leanings, and other demographic characteristics. This was followed by a thorough assessment of their personality traits as well as their sexual histories: How old were they when they lost their virginity? How many partners had they had altogether? Did they watch porn, and if so, how often? Had they ever been the victim of sexual abuse or assault? I also considered their overall sexual health status, including any current performance issues or concerns. As you'll soon see, asking all of these questions is what allowed me to get an in-depth look at what our fantasies say about who we are and where we are in our lives.

Finally, I asked participants how they typically appear in their own fantasies: Did they fantasize about themselves pretty much as they are, or did they give themselves a different personality, a different body type, maybe even change the appearance of their breasts or genitals? I also asked lots of questions about their fantasy partners, including whether they ever fantasized about celebrities and porn stars, or about their friends, or about fictional characters, even cartoon characters. And what did they do when they let their imaginations roam: Were they aroused by thoughts of kissing or oral sex, or did they want to engage in culturally taboo activities? And where the heck did their fantasies take place—in their bedrooms, at their offices, under a waterfall, out in the woods?

That's a lot to ask people about their sex lives—369 questions in total! But I did so with great care and concern for the well-being of the thousands of folks who graciously volunteered their time for this project. Before anybody took the survey, five experts—four psychologists and a medical doctor—reviewed it from start to finish. All information was collected anonymously to ensure participants' privacy and confidentiality, and it was collected with full informed consent—people knew what kinds of questions I would ask and what I would do with the answers they gave me.

Who Shared Their Fantasies with Me?

In total, 4,175 adults age eighteen or older who were current citizens or residents of the United States completed my survey, most of whom had heard about it through a major social media channel like Facebook, Twitter, or Reddit. Given that this was the primary way people learned about my survey, the demographics of my sample tended to skew more toward the average social media user than they did toward the average American. For instance, the median age of my survey participants (thirty-two) was about six years younger than the overall median age in America.[3] Likewise, my participants were more highly educated and more affluent than the average American. My survey did not disproportionately attract people of one sex, though—it was virtually a fifty-fifty split between those who said they were born male and those who were born female.

Most of my participants said they were heterosexual (72 percent); however, sizable numbers identified as bisexual (12.6 percent), gay/lesbian (5.7 percent), pansexual (4.2 percent), or queer (2.3 percent). While this might make it sound like nonheterosexuals are vastly overrepresented in my survey, some recent national surveys have found that as many as one-third of adults under age thirty say they aren't completely heterosexual.[4] When you combine people's increasing willingness to adopt alternative sexual identity labels with the slightly younger skew of my sample, those percentages aren't as extreme as they might seem at first glance.

Because this survey called for uninhibited discussion of sexual fantasies, the people who chose to take part tended to have positive views about sex in general and were willing to openly report on their sex lives. As a result, it shouldn't be surprising to learn that religious folks and Republicans were somewhat underrepresented; however, many religious and political conservatives still ended up in my sample. Unfortunately, this recruitment issue is faced in virtually all sex research—people with conservative views about sex are simply less willing to sign up. Sex studies therefore tend to say a little more about people who are open to talking about sex and who are more comfortable with it. If anything, though, the kinds of people who did *not* take my survey are probably the ones who feel the most shame and guilt about their fantasies and are the least likely to have done anything about them. Thus, my results probably overestimate how many Americans have shared and acted on their sex fantasies.

Although my participants clearly had more positive views on sex than average, they weren't necessarily more sexually experienced than those who have taken part in nationally representative sex surveys. For instance, my participants didn't start having sex unusually early (they were in line with most everyone else, typically losing their virginity between ages fifteen and seventeen), they weren't having sex with an unusually high frequency (like most Americans, they were doing it somewhere between a few times per month and a few times per week), and they did not have an unusually high number of sex partners (my participants reported an average of eleven, which is right in line with recent numbers on the General Social Survey).[5] Most were involved in monogamous romantic relationships, too. Thus, while my participants may have viewed sex more positively than the average American, it wasn't the case that they had unusual sex lives.

While the demographics of my survey are not strictly representative of the US population, this is the largest and most diverse group of Americans that has ever been asked to report on their sexual fantasies. Almost all previous surveys on this topic have been limited exclusively to college students. Because my sample ultimately ended up including hundreds of Republicans, retirees, devoted religious followers, racial minorities, and persons who had not attended or graduated from college, I have the unprecedented ability to begin to shed light on what Americans from different walks of life are fantasizing about.

So Which Fantasies Are Americans' Favorites?

Once I'd collected all that data, I took a careful look at the single-word fantasy descriptions participants provided because I found them to be, well, utterly fascinating. The most popular words are shown in the word cloud below (the larger the word is, the more people used it to describe their favorite fantasy).

You may not be familiar with some of the words in this image, such as "cuckold" or "pegging"; however, if you keep reading, I promise to greatly expand your sexual vocabulary. As I looked through these words, I couldn't help but immediately notice some common trends, so I started to lump certain words to- gether into categories. For example, "threesome," "foursome," and "gangbang" were among the many words people used to de- scribe fantasies about sex with several people at the same time. So I put them together in the broader category of "multipart- ner sex." Likewise, "dominant," "submissive," "humiliation," and "restraint" were some of the words that helped shape a broader category called "power, control, and rough sex."

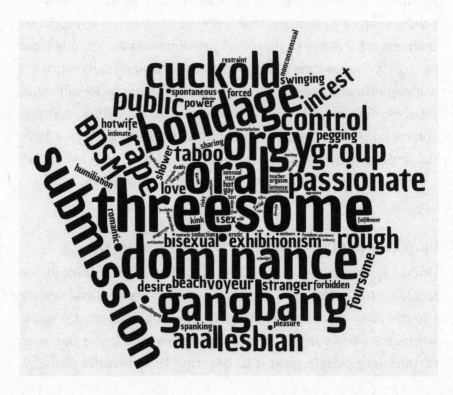

As I extracted these larger themes, I left out the words that were just too generic to be categorized, such as "sex" or "intercourse" (try harder next time, guys!). I also left out the incredibly esoteric ones that I had a really difficult time extracting a primary theme from, like "HumanCow." A heterosexual woman in her twenties made up this term to describe her desire to be tied up in the center of town and force-fed hormones that would make her lactate continuously so that she might be used as a human "milk machine" by thirsty townsfolk.

In the end, I extracted seven broader themes that accounted for the vast majority of all the fantasies submitted. Going from most to least common, they were:

1. multipartner sex
2. power, control, and rough sex
3. novelty, adventure, and variety
4. taboo and forbidden sex
5. partner sharing and nonmonogamous relationships
6. passion and romance
7. erotic flexibility—specifically, homoeroticism and gender-bending

To me, this collection of themes suggests that the American id is primarily characterized by desires to break free from cultural norms and sexual restraints. Most Americans have grown up learning that sex is only supposed to involve certain acts (penile-vaginal intercourse), that it is supposed to take place under very limited circumstances (within heterosexual, monogamous marriages), and that it's supposed to be done for utilitarian purposes (starting and growing a family). Our ids seem to be suggesting a variety of ways that we might rebel against those norms by trying out new, naughty, or downright taboo things.

Let's take a closer look at each theme. As we do, I'll recount several real fantasies. This will undoubtedly elicit a range of reactions among readers, from sexual arousal to laughter to shock to disgust. No matter your response, I encourage you to keep an open mind and continue reading. I guarantee that, if you do, you'll never think about sexual desire—your own or anyone else's—the same way again.

2

The Seven Most Common Sexual Fantasies in America

If You're Turned On by Any of This, You're in Good Company

Have you ever wondered whether your sexual fantasies are normal? If so, you've come to the right place. I'm going to answer that question for you in this chapter. But before I do, let me first establish what I mean by the term *normal*. As a scientist, saying that something is normal is basically the same as saying that something is statistically common. In other words, a normal fantasy is one that a lot of other people have. Just because a fantasy is normal doesn't mean it's healthy or appropriate to act on, though—that's an entirely separate issue, and one that we'll get into a little later. So, for now, let's just focus on which fantasies are normal in the sense of being common.

My analysis of Americans' favorite sexual fantasies revealed seven major categories that can be considered normal. If you've fantasized about these things before, chances are that you probably don't have anything to worry about—it's likely that your fantasies are pretty typical.

The Three Things That Almost Everyone Fantasizes About

We're going to begin by exploring the three most popular themes that emerged in my survey. These are the desires that almost everyone has had at one time or another, the things that, in all likelihood, your id has craved before. Following that, we'll discuss four additional themes, which are still common but not quite as pervasive. As we explore these themes, I'll offer some descriptions of each in the words of real people and point out the most interesting things I learned about them, as well as what science can tell us regarding the origins of these desires.

1. Multipartner Sex

The results of my investigation reveal that the single most popular sexual fantasy among Americans today is—drum roll, please—group sex. More than one-third of my participants described it as their favorite fantasy of all time, and when asked if they had *ever* fantasized about multipartner sex before—not just whether it was their favorite fantasy—the vast majority of both men and women agreed. In fact, it was rare for people to say they've *never* had such a fantasy—we're talking just 5 percent of men and 13 percent of women. In other words, group sex is perhaps the most normal thing there is to fantasize about because almost everyone has been turned on by the thought of it at one time or another.

So what do people imagine doing in a sex fantasy with multiple partners? There were really two main types of group sex fantasies I observed: those that involved threesomes, and those that involved a larger (usually unspecified) number of participants who took part in an orgy or gangbang.

"One, Two, Three... Peter, Paul, and Mary"

When it comes to group sex, three seems to be the magic number. In fact, "threesome" was, by far, the single most common term my participants used to describe their multipartner sex fantasies, and this was true for both men and women. Perhaps this is why Britney Spears's 2009 ode to threesomes (titled simply "3") topped the charts—more than just a catchy tune, this song's lyrics ("One, two, three... Peter, Paul, and Mary") echoed one of Americans' biggest pent-up erotic desires.

So who do Americans want to have threesome with? Do we tend to have specific people in mind, or does the appeal of a threesome simply reside more in what you can do—and see—when there's an extra person in bed? For their favorite fantasy of all time, I asked my participants to rate the importance of three different components of that fantasy: the activity that took place, the partner(s) involved, and the setting. What I found was that, for those who said group sex was their favorite fantasy, both men and women rated *what* they did as the most important aspect of this fantasy, and they rated it as being significantly more important than both *who* their partners were and *where* the event took place. It turned out that the partners themselves were rated as only moderately important, and the location as relatively unimportant. To me, what this suggests is that the appeal of threesomes has more to do with the fact that this activity creates a state of sensory overload than anything—it's really about amping up our arousal by bringing in another body that we can look at, touch, and experience in an overpowering way that allows us to get lost in sensations.

In light of this, it's probably not surprising that so many participants who had threesome fantasies described their partners generically. For example, as one straight guy in his twenties put it,

"Me and two very hot chicks in any and every position possible!!"
A lot of the threesome fantasies I received from men (gay and
straight alike) were similarly generic and succinct. By contrast,
women's group-sex fantasies tended to be a little more elaborate
(this wasn't surprising, given that women's fantasies in general
were more elaborate); however, I still found that many of the
women didn't spend any time at all detailing who their threesome
partners were, such as this straight woman in her forties who described her threesome fantasy in terms of an endurance contest
with two random dudes: "My greatest fantasy is to be with 2 men
at the same time. While one is fucking me the other is licking me.
Then they switch. Then I lay on the bed and they take turns fucking me but I will not let them cum. They both get to thrust into
me 5 times and then switch. They see who can go the longest
without cumming."

There were certainly some folks who cared more about who
their threesome partners were, though, and that included people who were in romantic relationships. Partnered individuals
often made their spouse or lover part of their ideal threesome,
which tells us that people who want threesomes aren't necessarily in troubled relationships, nor are they looking to replace their
partners—instead, they're usually looking to share an experience
together that everyone will enjoy. For example, one straight guy
in his thirties said his ultimate fantasy included both his wife and
his ex: "A threesome with my wife and a woman I used to have
wild sex with in college. It would be planned, beginning with
my wife and the other woman going down on each other and
using their mouths in other ways. I would watch. Then I would
be pulled in and have oral performed on me while going down
on one of the women. Sex would happen in multiple positions

and would finish with me cumming on the women's breasts and faces. They would then lick up the cum off each other." Likewise, a pansexual woman in her thirties included her partner in her threesome fantasy, but at the same time, she described the third person as a generic man: "Both my fiancé and I are bisexual, but I have rarely gotten the chance to see him in a sexual situation with another man since we've been together. My favorite thing to fantasize about is having a threesome with another bisexual man, and to watch him give and receive oral and anal sex. I almost always fantasize about having him inside me while another man is inside him, and all of us climaxing at the same time." This particular fantasy stood out to me because this woman described her partner as the center of attention in her ideal threesome. In most of the other threesome fantasies I received, people described themselves as being the center of attention, such as this heterosexual woman in her twenties, who made it explicitly clear that *she* would be the focal point: "I am part of a threesome with a man and another woman. I am engaging in reverse cowgirl with the man and the other woman is in front of me and between the man's legs, performing oral sex on me. The focus of this threesome is me, and not the man." It makes sense that most people want to be the center of attention in their threesome fantasy. For one thing, it's likely to increase feelings of personal validation— you're likely to feel more attractive and desired when you're getting most of the action. Plus, for those who feel a little insecure, being the center of attention would likely allay any potential concerns that your romantic partner is into someone else more than you. And then there's the fact that you're being pleasured by not just one but two people, which is going to feed into those feelings of sensory overload that I mentioned above.

One other interesting observation I made about threesome fantasies is that the gender ratio of the partners involved varied quite a bit. While some preferred scenarios featuring one woman and two men (WMM), others preferred two women and one man (MWW), and yet others preferred that everyone was the same sex (MMM or WWW). However, I noticed an important difference in the preferred gender ratio between men and women, a difference that has been noted by previous researchers.[1] Specifically, heterosexual men are far more likely to prefer MWW to WMM threesomes, whereas heterosexual women's interest in threesomes doesn't depend quite as much on the gender ratio. Put another way, straight women are more open to threesomes with a partner of the same gender. Heterosexual-identifying women are also more open to the idea of an entirely same-sex threesome than are straight men. Remember these findings, because they're the first of many that will come up in this book suggesting that women may be more erotically flexible than men when it comes to the gender of their partners.

Sex with Four or More

Of course, threesomes are just the tip of the iceberg when it comes to group sex, which Britney Spears alludes to at the end of her song "3": "Let's do it you and me… or three… or four on the floor." Some people fantasize about large numbers of partners, as in an orgy or gangbang. Although these sex acts weren't quite as popular as threesomes, the majority of both men and women I surveyed reported having had these kinds of group-sex fantasies before, too. They were similar to threesomes in the sense that most people fantasized about generic partners (unless they had a current romantic partner) and wanted to be the center of attention in these acts. However, they differed in that, in these larger groups, many people also described a desire to watch others have sex and/or "put on a show." Thus, there are some additional layers of stimulation to be had when sex takes place in a larger group setting.

2. Power, Control, and Rough Sex

Rivaling group sex for the most popular fantasy theme in America is bondage, discipline, dominance, submission, sadism, and masochism—or BDSM for short. I'll define all of these terms for you momentarily, but generally speaking, what we're talking about here are sexual desires that invoke themes of power, control, and/or rough sex. More than one-quarter of my participants described this as their favorite fantasy of all time, and even if it wasn't their all-time favorite, most people said they had fantasized about at least one BDSM act before. In fact, it was rare for people to not have any BDSM fantasies at all—just 4 percent of women and 7 percent of men had *never* had them. Clearly, BDSM—like group sex—is a very normal sexual desire, and as a result, it shouldn't be any surprise that a book and film series like *Fifty Shades of Grey* caught on.

Before we move on, I should say that it isn't uncommon for group-sex fantasies to incorporate elements of BDSM, especially in the case of gangbang fantasies, which typically feature one person being sexually dominated by several others. Thus, BDSM and multipartner sex often go hand in hand.

So what exactly is a BDSM fantasy? Upon hearing this term, many folks immediately conjure up an image of a medieval-looking dungeon full of torture devices of the worst kind. Although it's certainly the case that *some* BDSM practitioners do have (or want to have) their own dungeons and *some* of them may enjoy (or fantasize about enjoying) intense pain, it turns out that BDSM rarely takes this form in fantasy or in reality. BDSM actually refers to a very diverse set of practices, and they can range from mild to wild.

To better demonstrate what I mean, let me break down this acronym for you—but before I do, let me clarify that there is a lot of overlap between the different elements of BDSM and that people often fantasize about more than one type. In addition, keep in mind that what one desires when it comes to BDSM can change across contexts. This means, for example, that someone who fantasizes about being dominant in one setting might fantasize about being submissive in other settings, depending upon who their partner is and how they're feeling. To use the lingo of real-life BDSM practitioners, people who like to change up their role are known as *switches*.

B Is for Bondage

Bondage involves taking pleasure in the use of physical restraints. For example, some might take a cue from Christian Grey in *Fifty Shades* and bind their partner's hands with a necktie, whereas others might use handcuffs or shackles, and yet others might use a spreader bar (a rod that attaches to both ankles in order to keep the legs apart). What all of these activities have in common is that they involve one person surrendering control of his or her body to another, often with the intent of allowing him- or herself to be used as a sex object. For example, a pansexual woman in her thirties described her desire to be bound and used, but in a "loving" way: "Being tied up by my partner—they can do whatever they want to me. Though I'm completely under their control, they treat me lovingly and plea-sure me while I'm tied up. They use my body to get themselves off, but it's in a way that can only be described as lovingly." Of course, not everyone wants to be tied up—some want to tie up their partners, such as a straight man in his fifties who de-scribed his favorite fantasy as "my partner being tied up and I would be allowed to do everything that I can think of."

My survey results suggest that Americans like bondage. A lot. More than three-quarters of participants reported having had bondage fantasies before, and about one-third reported having them often. I suspect bondage is one of the most popular forms of BDSM in part because it's easy. It doesn't require a lot of skill or imagination, and you don't necessarily need any special equipment, either—I mean, we all have plenty of items in our closets that could work in a pinch. This is why bondage tends to be people's first stop in exploring BDSM, as well as a gate-way to more, ahem, advanced practices.

D Is for Discipline

Discipline is similar to bondage in that it involves deriving sex-ual arousal from the use of restraint; however, we're talking about *psychological* rather than physical restraint here. In other words, discipline is all about controlling someone else's behaviors—what they're allowed to do or say—through rules and punishment. As described by a straight woman in her for-ties: "I want to be controlled for my own good in a certain way, rewarded or denied reward based on my compliance."

Like bondage, discipline also involves one person surren-dering control to another; however, it is very different in that neither is playing a passive role—the partner who is being disciplined is an active participant who must comply with orders and commands, or else suffer (enjoy?) the consequences.

Discipline isn't quite as popular as bondage. Just over half of participants reported having discipline fantasies before, and about one-fifth reported having them often. Compared to bondage, discipline requires more active participation; you're not just a passive recipient of physical sensations but rather an actor who is playing a role. In some ways, then, discipline can be thought of as surrendering both body and mind to another. Not everyone is comfortable giving up quite so much control, which may help to explain why bondage tends to be a far more popular fantasy theme than discipline.

D Is Also for Dominance, While S Is for Submission

Dominance involves obtaining sexual pleasure from having power and control over another person, whereas submission involves receiving pleasure by ceding power and control to someone else. Please note that the "control" we're talking about here can be physical, psychological, or both, and that it may or may not involve bondage and/or discipline.

The submission fantasies I received took a lot of different forms, but they were fundamentally about giving oneself over completely to another person to be used for that person's pleasure. For example, one straight guy in his thirties described his desire to submit to a dominatrix as follows: "I have a fantasy of being sexually dominated by a woman. I want to be made to totally submit to her every need and desire. I want her to penetrate me with a strap-on. Be told to bend over and take it like a man. I want to be taken with a strap-on until she is exhausted. Then I want to be made to lick her all over until she orgasms."

Likewise, a bisexual woman in her late teens expressed the desire to submit to a man who will have his way with her: "Being put on a leash and forced to my knees, then a man writing words like 'slut' and 'whore' over my body, spitting on me, and forcing me to do whatever he wants me to do to him, calling me worthless and his slave." In both of these cases, the fantasy holder didn't just want to submit but to be humiliated in a way, too (e.g., being made to "take it like a man," being "forced to my knees," being branded "slut" or "whore"). What's the deal with that? Why do some people find humiliation to be a turn-on? It's likely because psychological pain has the same effects on us as physical pain, due to the fact that both of them activate the same areas of the brain.[2] One such effect is increased *mindfulness*, or feelings of being in the here and now. What this means is that pain, whether physical or psychological, makes us focus on our immediate sensations, and in doing so, it allows us to experience everything more intensely.[3] This means that if sexual stimulation follows some kind of pain—like being humiliated—you might find sex even more pleasurable than you otherwise would. It's akin to when you step in from the bitter cold and sip some hot cocoa—the pain of the cold makes your drink taste even more intense than usual.

The dominance fantasies I received were really interesting because the people who expressed them usually went out of their way to clarify that, while they wanted to dominate someone, they did not want to hurt them in any way. A bisexual woman in her thirties discussed the importance of caring for the men who are submissive to her: "My favorite sexual fantasy involves dominating two men. I always have control of what the men will do sexually. I engage freely in sexual activities with both men, and they both adore me and worship me. They both do whatever it takes to please me. I can have them both at the same time or they can even take turns. I tend to romanticize the aspect of having sex with two men at once by taking the role of the dominant who cares for her submissive men." As these examples illustrate, it seems that people with dominance fantasies recognize that power comes with responsibility and that those in the dominant role need to look out for the well-being of their submissive partners. In other words, dominance fantasies are *not* about a desire to harm someone else and, therefore, shouldn't necessarily be viewed as a sign of a pathological personality.

The vast majority of my participants reported fantasizing about both dominance and submission; however, more people reported submission fantasies, and they reported having them more often than those who had dominance fantasies. Thus, it seems that more Americans want to give up control rather than take control during sex. This might be, in part, because some don't want the responsibility that comes with taking control; however, it is likely also due to the fact that submission psychologically changes you from a person to an object and helps to take you out of your head. This is something that may be appealing to people who are easily distracted or tend to be anxious during sex.

S Is Also for Sadism, and M Is for Masochism

Finally, *sadism* and *masochism* refer to obtaining sexual pleasure from giving and receiving pain, respectively. Obviously, this can mean a number of different things depending upon one's personal preferences, from spanking and slapping to whipping and flogging to humiliation to putting clamps or clothespins on the nipples to dripping hot wax on the skin (as Madonna infamously did to Willem Dafoe in the Razzie Award–winning 1993 film *Body of Evidence*). Some live on the edge and elevate their pursuit of pain to dangerous and sometimes lethal levels by practicing activities like cutting, administering electric shocks, and undergoing oxygen deprivation (a practice that allegedly caused the death of actor David Carradine in 2009); however, these practices are relatively rare in both fantasy and reality. Most people who are into sadism and masochism report an interest in relatively mild pain that remains within consensual and very controlled limits and occurs in a context of mutual trust, care, and concern. For instance, this bisexual woman in her twenties described her favorite fantasy as "being spanked and dominated sexually.... Having someone who is loving in the care afterwards. Being tied down to a table in a kneeling position and being whipped and touched. Whatever the other person wanted to do within the limits."

Spanking, biting, and whipping were among the more commonly mentioned acts of sadomasochism in my survey. In describing these activities, participants were usually quick to clarify their limits: "gentle spanks," "forceful, but not aggressive," or "just rough enough... but not enough to inflict real pain." Some of my participants described desires for intense pain, including a few who said they wanted to be "beaten." For the most part, though, the ideal amount of pain seems to be in the mild to moderate range, enough to cause the desired effects in the moment—like increasing mindfulness—without leaving a mark or doing any kind of lasting damage.

Most of my survey participants reported having had both sadism and masochism fantasies. Generally speaking, however, it was more common for people to fantasize about receiving pain in some form than it was to fantasize about giving pain.

Fantasies About Forced Sex

One of the most common types of BDSM fantasies reported by my participants was forced sex. I've chosen to cover these fantasies in their own section for a few reasons. First, they are not easily categorized because they often cut across multiple areas of BDSM (in addition to themes of dominance-submission, they frequently include sadomasochistic elements and/or bondage at the same time). Beyond that, these fantasies are quite controversial and therefore deserve special attention.

Most of my participants with forced sex fantasies described them as "rape." Though that's the word they chose to use, it's probably not the most accurate one, given that these fantasies really tend to focus on token resistance and feature a scenario in which the fantasizer remains in complete control at all times and is not harmed. For example, a bisexual woman in her twenties described her forced-sex fantasy as follows: "I love it when my husband dominates me and it ends up escalating into a mock rape. It used to bother me to have this fantasy, due to the fact that I myself am a counselor and have worked both with rape victims and offenders. But after getting into my current relationship, I was able to explore a fantasy I never acted on in a safe, honest, and communicative relationship. And knowing that 'no' will still mean 'no' allows me to let go and enjoy the experience." As you can see, she describes her fantasy as "mock rape" and talks about the importance of safety and consent. Other participants included similarly important caveats, like "I know I'm safe and he knows my boundaries." These scenarios bear no resemblance to actual rape and instead are about a sex act that occurs on one's own terms.

Forced-sex fantasies are more common than you might think. In fact, nearly two-thirds of the women I surveyed reported having them. It's not just women who have forced-sex fantasies, though. More than half of the men I surveyed fantasized about being forced to have sex, too! Though women tend to have fantasies of this nature more often than men, they are not unique to one gender (or sexual orientation, for that matter).

It's worth mentioning that I received a handful of forced-sex fantasies that were quite intense. For instance, a straight woman in her twenties said: "I want to be naked, tied up, and humiliated. I want to be shown zero mercy. I want to be beat, slapped, and spanked like I deserve. I want my partner to force me to do anything he wants no matter what. I want him and 10 of his buddies to hate fuck me while I cry because I secretly enjoy it. I want to be bent over and taken in public....I want to feel like I am being raped and have absolutely no control and no say." I read thousands of fantasies in putting together this book, and this is among the few that have really stuck with me, because of the way this woman described wanting to get "hate fucked" and to be "shown zero mercy." If you found this language disturbing, you're not alone. However, if you read it carefully, it's clear that this woman (like everyone else with forced-sex fantasies) doesn't truly want to be raped, given that she talks about wanting to "feel like" she has no control and how she "secretly enjoys it." This scenario is only appealing to her because it takes place entirely in her head, where she remains in control the entire time.

To be clear, there is a spectrum when it comes to forced-sex fantasies, and the example included in the paragraph above comes from the most intense end. Therefore, it should not be viewed as representative. I simply mention it here to demonstrate how much variability there is in the content of forced-sex fantasies and how they sometimes include sadomasochistic elements, such as behaviors that make one feel degraded.

We'll return to the issue of forced-sex fantasies a bit later in the book because these fantasies pose some special safety concerns for those who wish to act them out with a partner.

3. Novelty, Adventure, and Variety

The third most popular sexual fantasy in America revolves around themes of novelty, adventure, and variety. Specifically, what I'm talking about here are: (1) sexual activities, like oral or anal sex, that one has never done before or would like to attempt in a new way; (2) having sex in unique settings, such as on the beach or in an airplane; and (3) having unexpected, surprising, or thrilling sexual encounters, such as getting it on in public or trying out a new sex toy. In other words, I'm talking about fantasies that take one's sex life in new and exciting directions. Fantasies like these were extremely common among my survey participants: about one in five described novelty as their favorite fantasy of all time, and far more said they fantasize about novelty on occasion.

Undoubtedly, there's some overlap here with fantasies about group sex and BDSM, both of which are appealing to many folks precisely because they represent a new or different way of having sex. However, it made sense to keep group sex and BDSM separate because it wouldn't do them justice to say that they're nothing but a yearning for novelty. As you'll see later on in this book, those fantasies have psychological origins and motives that go well beyond simply wanting to experiment with something different.

It's important to highlight that "novelty, adventure, and variety" is one of those things that means different things to different people. What's new and adventuresome for one person may be considered routine or dull by the next. Novelty is therefore one of the most diverse fantasy themes we'll consider. For ease of discussion, let's break this theme down into desires for new and exciting sexual activities and desires for sex in varied settings and locations.

Beyond the Missionary Position: Fantasies About Novel Sexual Activities

Like group sex and BDSM fantasies, the thing that turns most people on in novelty fantasies is the sexual act itself—what they're doing is usually more important than who their partner is or where it takes place. It therefore shouldn't be any surprise to learn that these fantasies tend to focus on things like oral and anal sex rather than the most traditional sex act of all: missionary-style penile-vaginal intercourse. Among my survey participants, there was certainly a lot of variability in which specific activities people wanted to engage in, but it was clear from a number of their descriptions that many were drawn to these acts simply because they weren't a part of their regular sexual routines. For example, one gay man in his forties summed up his favorite fantasy of all time simply as: "Oral sex, since I don't receive it."

Beyond oral and anal sex, participants described desires to switch up their usual intercourse positions. "Doggy style" was the most frequently mentioned position in Americans' favorite fantasies, and in general, it was men's favorite and women's second-favorite position to fantasize about, as you can see in the table below. Interestingly, both men and women fantasized more often about their partner being on top during intercourse rather than them, something that ties in well with the previously mentioned finding that people tend to fantasize more about being submissive than about being dominant (that, or maybe it's just a sign that a lot of Americans are lazy in bed).

The Intercourse Position Americans Fantasize About Most Frequently

	MEN	WOMEN
Position		
Doggy style	32.4%	33.3%
Face-to-face with you on top	21.6%	15.8%
Face-to-face with your partner on top	26.9%	38.2%
"Spooning" position	2.4%	2.3%
Reverse cowboy/cowgirl	7.7%	2.0%
Something else	7.7%	6.7%
Don't fantasize about intercourse	1.3%	1.7%

Beyond fantasizing about new sexual acts and positions, there are a lot of other ways people imagine adding variety to their sex lives. For instance, nearly 40 percent of participants reported having fantasized about experimenting sexually with food. I asked these folks which foods they usually think about, and, perhaps not surprisingly, whipped cream, chocolate, ice cubes, and strawberries were the foods of choice for most. The rest had some rather, um, interesting tastes, including blue cheese dressing, corn on the cob, dog food, and "gum from the

Willy Wonka movie." The least picky of my participants wrote in, "Anything that a man can ejaculate on and can be subsequently eaten."

Even more respondents (two-thirds) had fantasized about incorporating technology into their lovemaking. Of course, some fantasize about both food and tech, echoing the activities of *Seinfeld*'s George Costanza in a 1997 episode entitled "The Blood." George tried to achieve what he termed the "trifecta": having sex while watching a portable TV and chowing down on a pastrami sandwich. Unfortunately for George, it turned out that his girlfriend wasn't quite as into the idea as him because, well, he got a little too consumed by the other activities.

Playing sex games and sexual role-playing were other common ways people fantasized about adding variety, but perhaps the most popular—reported by 85 percent of participants—was using sex toys. BDSM props, such as blindfolds and handcuffs, were the toys most commonly mentioned in Americans' favorite fantasies, followed by strap-on dildos. Some may be surprised to learn that many women—gay, straight, and bisexual—said they had fantasized about wearing a strap-on and giving anal sex to someone else, while a lot of men—heterosexual and bisexual—said they had fantasized about receiving anal sex from a woman wearing a strap-on. This activity is known colloquially as "pegging," and there's sometimes a BDSM component to it, as you can see in the following fantasy submitted by a woman in her twenties who identified as "sexually fluid": "Currently one of my biggest sexual fantasies revolves around pegging—to be more specific, pegging a very masculine male. I find the idea of engaging in sexual activity with a masculine, large, muscular, submissive male, to be very hot." Why is pegging so popular? Part of the appeal is probably that it's a novelty in the sense that it goes against traditional gender roles, placing women in a dominant position and men in a submissive position; however, there's a bit more to it than that. Of course, the fact that it's taboo may make it appealing to some, but there's a biological explanation, too: anal sex can stimulate the male prostate gland (sometimes referred to as the P-spot), which many men find results in very powerful and intense orgasms.

It should be clear by now that Americans want their sex lives to be filled with diverse and varied activities. They don't just want to do one thing forever—they want to experiment and mix it up. As further evidence of this, check out the table below, which details the most common sexual activities Americans fantasize about and how they differ for men and women. The key things to note from these data are that (1) both men and women want a lot of variety in their sex lives, and (2) while there are obviously some differences in the numbers, there's actually a lot of commonality when it comes to the activities that men and women desire (the only exceptions being that men were a bit more likely to fantasize about sixty-nine-ing and giving anal sex). However, one especially fascinating thing to note from this table is the striking similarity between men and women with regard to fantasies about receiving anal sex—nearly two-thirds of each sex had fantasized about this before. Considering that my sample was predominately heterosexual (72 percent), this tells us that a heck of a lot of straight guys seem to be getting off on the idea of pegging and, presumably, P-spot orgasms. Of course, because I did not ask about *who* they wanted to receive anal sex from, some might interpret these results as a sign that some straight guys might not be quite as straight as they claim to be.

The Sex Acts Americans Fantasize About Most Frequently

	NEVER	SELDOM	SOMETIMES	OFTEN
KISSING				
Men	2.9%	11.5%	28.1%	57.4%
Women	2.5%	10.2%	18%	69.3%
MUTUAL MASTURBATION				
Men	9.9%	19.7%	34.9%	35.5%
Women	15.5%	23.9%	28.8%	31.8%
GIVING ORAL SEX				
Men	2.7%	6.5%	21.2%	69.6%
Women	5.9%	11.8%	25.2%	57.1%
RECEIVING ORAL SEX				
Men	3.0%	9.0%	21.5%	66.6%
Women	6.2%	12.6%	23.1%	58.1%
SIMULTANEOUS ORAL SEX (69)				
Men	10.6%	18.9%	28.8%	41.7%
Women	32.5%	26.2%	19.7%	21.6%
VAGINAL INTERCOURSE				
Men	6.9%	5.2%	12.6%	75.4%
Women	1.4%	2.7%	12.2%	83.7%
GIVING ANAL SEX (WITH A PENIS OR STRAP-ON)				
Men	19.0%	18.8%	25.3%	36.9%
Women	60.4%	20.3%	12.3%	7.0%
RECEIVING ANAL SEX				
Men	41.9%	20.6%	18.1%	19.5%
Women	38.9%	19.3%	22.7%	19.2%
USING SEX TOYS				
Men	15.9%	21.1%	35.9%	27.0%
Women	14.0%	20.2%	34.5%	31.3%

Beyond the Bedroom: Fantasies About Sex in Varied Settings

Novelty and adventure aren't only about trying new sexual acts and positions—after all, the human body can only contort in so many ways (Cirque du Soleil performers notwithstanding). As a result, many of us seek to inject novelty and adventure into our sex lives by performing our favorite acts somewhere other than in our own bed. Although it's not quite as important as the sex act itself, I found that the setting was still a very important component of many people's novelty fantasies—and in fact, my participants said that the setting was a more important element in their novelty fantasies than it was in their group sex and BDSM fantasies.

As I read through my participants' favorite fantasies, "public" emerged as the preferred setting. "Public" can, of course, mean a lot of things, but for some folks, the specific location doesn't really matter as long as they are having sex in a place where other people are (or could be) around. However, some folks did include very specific public locations in their fantasies—most commonly, places like an office, bathroom, elevator, bar, locker room, or park. Most of these fantasies about public sex seemed to be driven by the same thing: a sense of adventure and the thrill that one could potentially be observed or caught in the act. Many of my participants explicitly said something to this effect, including a straight man in his fifties who described his favorite fantasy as "making love to a stranger in a semi-public place with a risk of being discovered." A straight woman in her thirties expressed similar sentiments: "Sex in public. In a slightly private area but with some chance of exposure, like an empty courtyard."

As these examples reveal, people with public-sex fantasies don't necessarily want others to watch them have sex—they just want there to be a risk of it happening. In this sense, these fantasies are very different from exhibitionism fantasies or scenarios in which people truly want to put on a show (we'll get to those shortly). Public-sex fantasies are therefore more about enhancing sex by inducing an element of risk and fear than anything else. This makes sense in light of a large body of research finding that people have a tendency to mistake strong emotions—like fear and anger—for sexual arousal.[4] Why is that? It's because these emotions stimulate our bodies, causing our hearts to beat faster and our breathing to become heavier, among other things. Although these bodily changes aren't sexual per se, it's easy for us to mistakenly interpret them as such, especially if they occur in the presence of a powerful sexual stimulus, such as someone you think is pretty hot. For example, heterosexual men who are asked to jog in place for a few minutes (and therefore amp up their physiological arousal levels) prior to evaluating the attractiveness of a female stranger find her to be sexier than heterosexual men who are sedentary.[5] In other words, the exercisers' feelings of arousal seem to transfer to the stranger in a way that intensifies their overall feelings of attraction toward her. The key idea here is really that if we fantasize about sex in a setting that evokes a lot of strong emotions—such as doing it in public—it has the potential to produce a far more intense state of sexual arousal than the thought of sex in a less novel location, like your own bed.

Beyond public settings, the next most common locations people mentioned in their favorite fantasies were—in order—on a beach, outdoors or in nature, and in the shower. In fantasies about beach and nature settings, participants were often (but not always) quick to clarify that these areas were meant to be remote or secluded, indicating that it's not so much about the risk of discovery but more about how the setting itself makes them feel—free, relaxed, sensual, romantic—and how that enhances the sex. One straight man in his forties summed up this idea perfectly: "One of my main fantasies would be to be outdoors—the wind blowing on our bodies, very stimulating. No fear of getting caught at all." Interestingly, he didn't even mention sex in this fantasy—it was almost an afterthought! Women's fantasies about novel settings tended to be a bit more elaborate, taking a lot of time to set the scene. For example, one straight woman in her twenties told me her fantasy involved "walking on the beach during a warm summer night. The beach is empty and there is just me and my partner breathing the sea air. We have a bottle of champagne that is still crisp. We lay down directly on the sand and we begin looking at each other. Then we start taking off each other's clothes while aggressively making out. Then we start making love and do it throughout the whole night." This particular fantasy is a great example of one in which the setting has a profound effect: the warmth of the summer air, the scent of the ocean, and the taste of the champagne all come together to create a multisensory experience that enhances the sex. If you think about it, fantasies like this are really aimed at producing the same mental state that many BDSM practitioners are after: mindfulness, or being in the here and now. These elaborate fantasy settings are all about promoting relaxation and eliminating distractions in a way that allows one to more intensely experience both sex and the environment in which it takes place.

I asked my participants how often they had fantasized about sex in a number of specific locations and discovered that most people fantasize about having sex in multiple places. More than three-quarters reported fantasizing about sex in exotic locales (beaches and waterfalls), bodies of water (hot tubs, swimming pools, and showers), nature (forests and fields), hotels, and motor vehicles. Fewer, but still a majority, reported fantasizing about sex in highly public settings, such as in the workplace, at school, in a library, and on an airplane. People who fantasized about any one of these settings were more likely to have fantasized about the others, which suggests that settings are simply more important or desirable to some people.

So What Do These Three Types of Fantasies Have in Common?

What ties together the three major fantasy themes we've discussed thus far is that they're all fundamentally about changing things up when it comes to sex—varying partners, sensations, activities, and settings. It makes perfect sense that fantasies about sexual variety are so popular in light of a mountain of research finding that our arousal tends to habituate or lessen over time in response to the same sexual stimulus. In order to get the juices flowing again, so to speak, we need to mix things up. This observation has been dubbed the Coolidge Effect, borrowing its name from a popular anecdote about former president Calvin Coolidge and his wife, Grace.[6] The story goes something like this: the first couple visited a chicken farm together, and on their guided tour, the president trailed a bit behind his wife. While visiting the hen yard, Mrs. Coolidge took note of one particularly potent rooster that went from one hen to the next. She asked the tour guide to be absolutely sure to point out that rooster to the president when he came by. The guide obliged. When President Coolidge arrived at the yard, he was informed of the rooster's sexual prowess and, further, that his wife was the one who thought it should be brought to his attention. The president paused for a moment and responded, "Tell Mrs. Coolidge that there is more than one hen."

Scientists have documented the Coolidge Effect by looking at what happens when people watch the same exact porn clip each day for a week or longer. What researchers typically find is that both men and women exhibit less arousal the more frequently they see the same erotic material.[7] By changing things up, not only can we reverse this trend, but we can potentially have more powerful orgasms, too. In one study, researchers asked straight men to masturbate to scenes from the same porno featuring the same two actors over a period of two weeks.[8] (Incidentally, I can only imagine the effect this study must have had on participants' social lives: "I'm sorry, but I can't go out tonight. I need to masturbate. For science.") When these guys were finally given a new porn clip to watch at the end of the study (one in which the only real difference was that it involved a new actress), these men didn't just ejaculate faster but also produced semen containing a greater number of active sperm. In other words, it seems that straight guys actually become more sexually potent upon seeing a new attractive woman!

So what's behind the so-called Coolidge Effect, anyway? Increasingly, scientists believe there's an evolutionary explanation, with some arguing that perhaps the Coolidge Effect evolved in order to support a nonmonogamous approach to mating. Think of it this way: being titillated by novelty decreases the odds that we'd pass up perfectly good mating opportunities. We can't say for sure that this is why the Coolidge Effect exists, but the fact that it exists at all can help explain why so many of us find things like group sex, BDSM, and novel scenarios to be arousing: they offer just the kind of variety necessary to kick-start waning levels of sexual desire and solve our habituation problem.

The Big Three Fantasies and the American Id

The three major things the American id is craving are sex with multiple partners, BDSM, and sexual adventure/variety. As you've seen, each of these fantasies can take many forms, but certain forms are more desired than others. For instance, when it comes to multipartner sex, threesomes are preferred to orgies and gangbangs. With BDSM, Americans seem to want to spend a bit more time on bondage, submission, and masochism than they do on dominance and sadism. And when it comes to adventure/variety, Americans seem to care a little more about trying new sexual positions and activities than they do about having sex in new settings.

Any way you look at it, though, if you're fantasizing about these types of things, you're in good company, because almost everyone else is, too—due at least in part to the Coolidge Effect. However, these are far from the only kinds of fantasies that could be considered "normal" (in the sense of being statistically common). As I read through the thousands upon thousands of fantasies that I received, four other important themes emerged. Although they were less common than the big three fantasies, they were certainly still popular and clearly reflect other normative elements of the American id. So what kinds of desires are we talking about? Let's take a look.

Four Other Kinds of Fantasies that Are Absolutely, Completely, Totally Normal

Three of the next four fantasies we'll consider are tied together by a common thread: breaking the rules. These are the things that we're most definitely not supposed to want, at least according to the modern moral and political authorities in America. Forget lifelong monogamy, heterosexuality, and vanilla sex—the American id wants to test our sexual boundaries and limits.

At the same time, though, the id has its gentler, more romantic side: Americans also crave passion and intimacy with the ones they love. We want to feel that sense of irresistible attraction to our partners—the kind where you and your lover literally can't keep your hands off of each other. But we want to feel an emotional, sometimes spiritual connection to our partners as well. So it's certainly not the case that our ids are one-note, inevitably calling out for sexual debauchery—they are also yearning for romance and comfort. Let's start by talking about the debauchery, though. After all, it was a bit more popular.

4. Taboo and Forbidden Sex

Most of us have fantasized at one time or another about "forbidden fruit"—sexual activities that are considered taboo by our culture, society, or religion. In some ways, these fantasies are an extension of the novelty and adventure fantasies we discussed earlier; however, the specific sexual desires we'll consider here are distinctly different from run-of-the-mill novelty fantasies in the sense that (1) taboo desires are more likely to be considered disgusting (like licking someone else's feet); (2) some of these desires, like voyeurism and exhibitionism, would be illegal to act upon; and (3) almost all of these desires have been formally classified as paraphilias by the mental health community.

As we've already established, the term *paraphilia* necessarily implies that a given sexual interest is "uncommon" or "unusual"; however, my survey results suggest that taboo desires are actually pretty widespread. In fact, in my analysis of Americans' favorite fantasies of all time, taboo activities emerged more often than did fantasies of love and romance! In addition, when asked whether they've *ever* fantasized about a number of different taboo and forbidden activities, most of my participants reported doing so at least once before. This isn't to suggest that *all* taboo desires are common, though. The more deviant and extreme the desire, the rarer it tends to be. So what we're going to focus on here are the three most common taboos that Americans get off on thinking about.

A Room with a View: Peeping Toms and Nosy Rosies

By far, the most common taboo activity Americans fantasize about is voyeurism. What we're talking about here is the desire to watch other people undress or have sex *without* their knowledge or consent. Believe it or not, most of my participants (60 percent) reported having fantasized about this before! The point of voyeurism fantasies is to observe others without being seen. For example, one straight man in his fifties described his voyeurism fantasy as "being unnoticed and anonymously watching beautiful naked women masturbating." "Spying" would therefore be another way to think about this.

Voyeurs imagine a wide range of scenarios. They include everything from snooping on other people's sexual exploits through hidden video cameras (like Billy Baldwin's character did in the 1993 erotic thriller *Sliver*) to watching people undress through a peephole in the wall (à la Norman Bates in Alfred Hitchcock's classic film *Psycho*) to being invisible and sneaking into people's bedrooms (as Kevin Bacon's character did in the sci-fi flick *Hollow Man*).

To be clear, voyeurism isn't about becoming aroused in response to any and all visual sexual stimuli. Therefore, people who like to make love with the lights on, who enjoy visiting strip clubs, and who watch a lot of porn aren't really displaying voyeuristic behavior. True voyeurism is nonconsensual in nature because it involves someone being spied upon without their awareness. Given that consent is lacking in these cases, voyeurism is illegal when the fantasy becomes reality.

Although it's very common for people to have fantasized about voyeurism at least once before, not many people fantasize about it often. Most people prefer partnered, physical encounters to this more solitary activity. Most of us don't want to risk being arrested, either. Research suggests that those who have voyeurism fantasies regularly tend to have difficulties establishing conventional sexual relationships, which tells us that very frequent voyeurism fantasies may be a sign that one has a deficit when it comes to sexual and/or romantic skills.[9]

Feet and Panties and Boots, Oh My! The Surprisingly Popular World of Fetish Fantasies

Fetishes are another popular taboo that appears in many Americans' sexual fantasies. In fact, nearly half of the Americans I surveyed (45 percent) reported that they fantasize about fetish objects—objects that one relies on for feelings of sexual arousal. When this object is present during sex or masturbation, one typically has an easier time becoming and staying aroused and reaching orgasm. Some fetishes are very mild, meaning that the object isn't absolutely necessary for one to enjoy sex. However, other fetishes are more intense, in the sense that one's ability to become aroused and enjoy sex just isn't the same in the absence of that fetish object.

People can have fetishes for virtually anything. Among the more unusual ones I've read about are cars, dirt, and medical devices (including, surprisingly enough, pacemakers—I wonder, is there an element of BDSM to this one?). More commonly, fetishes tend to involve articles of clothing, such as stockings, shoes, boots, or panties (sometimes well-used panties, like the contraband undies Piper Chapman peddles from prison in *Orange Is the New Black*). People with fetishes may wear, look at, fondle, and/or smell their preferred item during sex. For example, a straight man in his forties described his favorite fantasy to me as masturbating while watching a woman model Lycra pantyhose: "My biggest fantasy has no intercourse involved. I place an ad in Craigslist looking for a woman who enjoys watching a man masturbate. The only catch is when she gets to my apartment, she puts on control top pantyhose, preferably made from Lycra. She doesn't have to get nude, she can have a bra and panties on underneath. Or even a t-shirt. As she's sliding her legs into the hose, I'm masturbating. After she's done adjusting, she poses for me and encourages me to cum." The question many of you are probably asking after reading this fantasy is, "Why Lycra?" Well, Lycra (or, as it's more commonly known, spandex) is a very form-fitting fabric that essentially creates a second skin—you can still see someone's body shape and features underneath it. Lyrca is one of the most common fabrics people develop fetishes for because it doesn't hide anything, it can enhance the appearance of certain body parts (such as by making legs looking thinner and smoother), it has a unique texture, and people associate it with the genitals, since stockings, swimsuits, and underwear are often made from this material. The latter reason is probably why articles of clothing like bras and panties (regardless of material) tend to be among the most common fetish objects—they're endowed with erotic significance by virtue of the fact that they come into contact with the breasts and genitals.

Body parts that aren't typically a focus of sexual desire—things other than penises, breasts, vulvas, and butts—represent another common fetish object. Among the more common body parts that people sexualize are feet. In fact, one in seven survey participants reported having had a fantasy before in which feet or toes played a prominent role. For example, one "mostly straight" guy in his late teens described his fantasy in terms of touching, smelling, and licking other men's feet: "We both lie in the bed naked. He suddenly, slowly moves his feet towards my face. We talk a little bit while I slowly massage his feet. I take multiple whiffs of his feet. He laughs, and I start to lick his soles and his toes." Beyond feet, some find stomachs or abs, belly buttons, hands, or armpits to be sexually arousing. I should also clarify that breasts, genitals, and butts can rise to the level of fetish objects when people find that (1) they are *only* turned on by these body parts and (2) these body parts need to take on a very specific appearance in order to stimulate arousal. Think of straight guys who only go for women with extra-wide rear ends (as in, baby *really* got back), as well as straight women and gay men who only go for dudes with massive penises (the "size queen" fetish, as it has been dubbed in popular culture).

Where do fetishes come from? Most fetishes seem to be learned, in the sense that the people who have them can often tie their interests back to a very specific sexual experience in which their fetish object happened to be present when they had a very intense orgasm. This is something psychologists call *one-trial learning*, which refers to the idea that sometimes we learn associations between a stimulus and response on the very first try.

Something that contributes to this learning process is the fact that new sexual experiences are, in a way, giving us new types or kinds of orgasms that differ from those that came before.[10] This occurs because new sensations—things that we can see, smell, taste, hear, or feel—are modulating how aroused we are in that moment and how pleasurable the experience is. The sensations that we come to associate with greater pleasure and better orgasms then go on to become the focus of our sexual desires. Another way to think about this is that when it comes to sex, we don't necessarily know in advance what we're going to like until we try it. When we discover new sensations that we particularly enjoy, it can end up adjusting our threshold for orgasm and, ultimately, what we desire in future sexual encounters.

But how does that explain why we sometimes come to associate things with sex that gross a lot of people out, like feet? The other important part of this story is that sexual arousal reduces our disgust impulses, meaning that when we're horny, the things we normally find to be gross don't seem quite as bad. Consider a study in which young heterosexual men were asked to rate the appeal of twenty different sexual stimuli under two conditions: once while they were masturbating, and again while in an unaroused state.[11] The stimuli included a lot of things most people think are disgusting, from sex with animals to watching a woman urinate. Subjects rated these stimuli on a laptop in a private room. (The laptop was covered in plastic wrap to protect it from any, ahem, accidents.) Participants in the masturbation condition were explicitly told not to ejaculate and instead to maintain a "sub-orgasmic level of arousal." In the end, it turned out that nineteen of the twenty stimuli were rated as more attractive in the masturbation condition. In other words, when these guys were aroused, almost everything and everyone seemed more attractive to them.

The question you're probably wondering about is *why*—why would sexual arousal change our disgust response? Perhaps because sex itself can be a little messy. Some scientists believe that this is an evolutionarily adaptive response because toning down our disgust impulses might help to ensure that we don't miss out when a good chance to reproduce comes our way. The unintended side effect, though, is that it opens the door to developing all kinds of fetishes and unusual sexual interests. It also helps to explain why so many people feel ashamed of themselves after they reach orgasm while watching porn—their disgust response kicks in before they can close all of their open internet browser tabs. I suspect this is why the Command-Option-W shortcut on Macs was invented.

Putting on a Show: Exhibitionism Fantasies

Following closely on the heels of fetishism in popularity was exhibitionism, which involves exposing one's genitals or engaging in a sex act while others look on. There are really two types of exhibitionism that differ based on the desired reaction of others to what you're, um, "exhibiting": Do they want to see it, in which case they'll enjoy the show? Or are you planning to take them by surprise, in which case they'll likely be shocked or offended? The former—consensual exhibitionism—was about four times more common among my survey participants than the latter, nonconsensual type (42 percent and 10 percent, respectively). This suggests that, in most exhibitionism fantasies, the goal is not to violate or offend onlookers—rather, the hope is that others will like what they see, such as in the scenario this straight female participant in her thirties described: "My male partner and I are in a storefront of a building on a very busy street. Instead of a window, it is a one-way mirror (people can see in, we can't see out). We're having sex while unknown passersby stop to watch."

Consensual exhibitionism fantasies are similar to the public-sex fantasies we previously discussed. However, whereas those public-sex fantasies emphasized arousal from the prospect that one could *potentially* be observed, the fantasies we're talking about here focus on people who know for a fact that they *are* being observed. In other words, consensual exhibitionism isn't about arousal from the fear that one might be caught but rather arousal from knowing that others are watching—and taking pleasure in what they're seeing. So there's a certain amount of pleasure derived here from the simple knowledge that others think you're hot.

Nonconsensual exhibitionism is quite different in that it's necessarily illegal when this fantasy becomes reality because those who are observing aren't willing participants. As was the case with frequent voyeurism fantasies, those who have a strong desire for nonconsensual exhibitionism tend to have difficulties establishing conventional relationships and may be lacking in social skills.[12]

5. Swinging, Partner Sharing, and Polyamory

Related to the previous category of taboo and forbidden sexual desires are fantasies about nonmonogamous relationships— relationships in which people are free to pursue more than one sexual and/or romantic partner at the same time. Given that monogamy is the norm in modern America, departures from it tend to be considered deviant. Of course, nonmonogamy fantasies also overlap with multipartner fantasies in that they are fundamentally about having more than one sex partner. However, the difference is that nonmonogamy fantasies don't necessarily involve several people having sex *as a group;* rather, they're about having a relationship in which the partners agree that certain forms of outside sexual activity are acceptable.

Most people who have nonmonogamy fantasies are in monogamous relationships themselves. For the most part, these folks want to keep their partners; however, they want to augment their relationships by bringing other sexual and/or romantic partners into the mix. Most people want to do this *consensually*, though, meaning these fantasies aren't necessarily about infidelity per se. Instead, in nonmonogamy fantasies, one's partner has provided their consent or blessing. Also, it may surprise you to learn that these folks aren't just fantasizing about being nonmonogamous themselves; they may fantasize about their partners being nonmonogamous as well—and sometimes a partner's nonmonogamy is an even bigger turn-on.

Like all of the other fantasy themes we've considered so far, nonmonogamy fantasies can take many forms; again, though, these fantasies reflect an element of mutual consent more often than not. In fact, fantasizing specifically about nonconsensual nonmonogamy—that is, cheating and infidelity—was actually quite rare when I combed through my participants' favorite fantasies of all time: less than one-half of 1 percent specifically described their favorite fantasy of all time as "cheating," "infidelity," or "adultery." By contrast, it was almost ten times more common for people to say their favorite fantasy reflected some form of consensual nonmonogamy (CNM). Likewise, when I looked at whether participants had *ever* fantasized about cheating or certain forms of CNM, like, say, having an open relationship or being polyamorous, both men and women were far more likely to say they'd fantasized about the latter. This suggests that Americans find the prospect of mutually agreeable nonmonogamy much more arousing than the secretive and deceptive kind.

So what does a CNM fantasy look like? Being in an open relationship was the most common form this fantasy took (79 percent of men and 62 percent of women had fantasized about it before). In an open relationship, the partners consent to a set of rules that allow one or both of them to pursue sex with others. As described by a straight man in his forties, "I repeatedly fantasize about being in an open relationship with my wife. Whether it is her or I with other people, either strangers or acquaintances, this is my biggest fantasy that I've never shared with her." As this example illustrates, what we're really talking about here are relationships in which people maintain one long-term romantic partner, but each person has some amount of outside sexual freedom.

Polyamory was the next most commonly fantasized about form of CNM, reported by 51 percent of women and 70 percent of men. Polyamory is different from being in an open relationship in the sense that the partners agree to have multiple sexual and/or romantic relationships simultaneously. Thus, polyamorous individuals may maintain several intimate, committed relationships at the same time. For example, a straight man in his forties described his favorite fantasy as "a full polyamorous relationship where all parties are both emotionally and physically compatible and involved."

Following open relationships and polyamory in popularity was swinging, which 66 percent of men and 45 percent of women said they had fantasized about. This refers to the desire to temporarily exchange or swap romantic partners, such as when two heterosexual married couples swap spouses for an evening. Other swingers engage in *full swap*, in which each person involved has sex with everyone else, regardless of gender, such as in this fantasy submitted by a man in his thirties who identified as "mostly straight": "I am bisexual, but only interested in a physical relationship with another man. I fantasize about fulfilling this with a full swap with my wife and another couple. Obviously, the other man would need to be bi as well."

Some swingers prefer for everyone to have sex in the same room during the swap because they find it arousing to watch their partners receive pleasure from others and/or because they want to make more than one swap. However, others are unsure of how they'd feel about seeing their partners have sex with someone else, like this straight man in his thirties: "My top fantasy is swinging. I don't know if I would feel comfortable or not seeing my wife with other men, nor do I think she would enjoy seeing me with other women. However, the thought of open sex between a group of friends is highly arousing."

Related to swinging is a practice in which people agree to let their partners have sex with other people, as long as they can watch it happen or at least hear about it later. In colloquial terms, this is known as *cuckolding* or *cuckqueaning*, depending upon whether the observer/listener is male or female. In psychological terms, it is known as *troilism*, and it has been classified as a paraphilia.

Interestingly, a majority of men who took my survey (58 percent) reported having had this fantasy before, and more than a quarter of them said they fantasize about it often, suggesting that, at least for men, this is far from rare or unusual, as the paraphilia label implies. These fantasies were a bit less common among women (just over one-third of female participants reported having them), but they certainly weren't unheard-of.

The men I surveyed were more likely to fantasize about their partners having sex with others than they were to fantasize about having sex while their partners looked on. For women, however, the reverse was true. This suggests that men and women find different roles more arousing in cuckolding scenarios. To illustrate this idea, consider this fantasy submitted by a man in his fifties who identified as "mostly straight": "I would like to see my wife from a distance sitting at a bar in a classy restaurant and being picked up by a complete stranger. They would make out a little before leaving the restaurant and then—after having the most amazing sex—come back. He goes his way, after which my wife joins me at the table where I was sitting in the first place. Then we get into our car and make love and have steaming sex before we go home." In this case, the man didn't necessarily even want to see the sex his wife was having—he just wanted to know it had taken place. Most of the guys I surveyed wanted to watch their partners in the act, but for some, it clearly wasn't essential.

By contrast, consider this scenario, submitted by a straight woman in her thirties: "I am currently living out my sexual fantasy in my marriage. A mutual friend of ours comes over at least once per week and fucks me hard while my husband sits in the corner, watches me, and strokes himself. It is so hot. I love having the confidence to stare in my husband's eyes and tell him how great my lover's cock feels as he is thrusting in and out of me." Most of the women I surveyed who reported fantasies about cuckolding described scenarios along these lines, in which they had sex while their partners watched or they simply told their partners about it after the fact. However, there were a few women who wanted their partners to go out and have sex with others, like this straight woman in her forties who said: "I love watching my husband have sex with other women. I like to be a part of the start of the relationship through to the sex and have sex with my husband after he's been with another woman. I don't get jealous and nothing arouses me more. If I don't get to watch, I love him to describe his encounter in graphic detail as we have sex."

As you may have noticed, cuckolding fantasies often feature elements of submission and masochism, and this appears to be especially true in heterosexual relationships where the man plays the role of observer. In these fantasies, the man is often humiliated, sometimes for having a small penis, such as in this scenario submitted by a straight man in his fifties:

I have an intense and long lasting fantasy that my wife would have sex with other men, or even have a boyfriend whom she has sex with often. Of course he has a larger cock than me and she really enjoys it all. When she comes home she allows (or "requires") me to go down on her and suck his cum from her. She really gets off on that and cums again from that. After she cums a few times from my tongue, she lets me fuck her. She

tells me how much bigger his cock is, and how much better he
is, of course.

In heterosexual men's cuckolding fantasies, the men are
ceding all power and control to their wives or girlfriends and
taking on a rather submissive and sometimes masochistic role.
This frequent overlap with BDSM makes cuckolding stand out
from other nonmonogamy fantasies.

Although open relationships, polyamory, swinging, and cuckolding are all practiced very differently, they do share some
similarities in terms of their psychological origins. Of course, all
of these forms of nonmonogamy can potentially be explained
through the lens of the Coolidge Effect in the sense that they
offer sexual variety and therefore help fend off habituation
of arousal. However, they can also be explained through *self-
expansion theory*, the idea that humans have a need to continually grow and expand the self in order to be satisfied with
their lives.[13] We can meet this need by having new experiences,
learning new things, and developing new relationships. From
this perspective, then, fantasies about consensual nonmonogamy can be viewed as an outgrowth of our ongoing quest for
self-expansion. An alternative way to think about this is that
monogamy has a tendency to thwart self-expansion because
monogamous sex can easily become predictable and stale if the
partners aren't careful. Consensual nonmonogamy allows one
to maintain a valued relationship while also introducing an avenue for continually fulfilling one's expansion needs.

In contrast to the consensual nature of open relationships,
polyamory, swinging, and cuckolding, some people fantasize
about straight-up infidelity or adultery. However, among those

who described this as their favorite fantasy of all time, the arousing part seemed to be the thrill of sneaking around or potentially being caught more than anything else, such as this bisexual woman in her late teens described: "I'm cheating on my boyfriend with my coworker while waiting for my boyfriend to come home so we have to be quick and it has to be dirty and fast." For others, the appeal of cheating fantasies is more about doing something "bad," such as this "mostly straight" woman in her twenties told me: "Having an affair with an often older, married, influential man. I just like the idea of doing something wrong and immoral—perhaps even a little 'gross' because they have many more years on me. I don't really fantasize about living with or being in the life of this man—I basically just want him around for me to tease and have sex with whenever I want. Plus the allure of sneaking around is attractive to me." As you can see, compared to CNM fantasies, infidelity fantasies appear to have quite different motivations behind them. Infidelity fantasies seem to have more in common with the adventure/variety and taboo fantasies we discussed earlier.

6. Intimacy, Romance, and Passion

By this point, you might be tempted to think that Americans' favorite sexual fantasies can be reduced to the following: trying new and kinky sex acts with multiple partners. However, there's far more to our fantasies than this. Americans definitely have a lot of fantasies that revolve around passion, intimacy, and romance, too.

The fantasies we'll consider in this section are quite different from the others we've seen thus far in that they typically have a strong emphasis on emotional fulfillment. This can include everything from just wanting to feel desired to sharing a deep, intimate connection with another person. In other words, these fantasies go well beyond simply gratifying a sexual urge—they also help us to meet profound emotional needs, especially something called *the need to belong*.[14] Social psychologists believe that human beings have a fundamental need to develop and maintain strong social connections throughout their lives. This need is second only to basic survival needs—things like thirst, hunger, and safety. It's really *that* important. In fact, when our need to belong isn't met, our physical health and psychological well-being deteriorate. And if we go for a prolonged period of time without meeting this need for social connection, there could potentially even be implications for how long we live. We can meet our need to belong in many ways, including through our families, friends, and coworkers. However, perhaps the single most important way we can do this is through our romantic and sexual relationships. In fact, for many people, romantic partners are their ultimate source of need fulfillment, which is why losing a partner to death or divorce can be so devastating. In light of this, fantasies about emotionally connecting with a partner can largely been seen as an outgrowth of this very powerful need to belong—the need to establish, or in some cases reestablish, a strong social connection.

Perhaps not surprisingly, desires for intimacy and emotional connection tend to be tied to particular people, as opposed to, say, just another hot body with a generic face. The specific partner involved in these fantasies is often just as important—if not more so—than the sexual activity that's taking place. What may surprise you, though, is that fantasies about meeting emotional needs don't live up to gender stereotypes. Fantasies about being desired, validated, loved, and bonded to a partner are common

among both women *and* men—and in part, that's because the
need to belong is not something that's specific to one gender.

What's Love Got to Do with It?

Among my survey participants whose favorite fantasy of all time
reflected this theme, the most common words used to describe
it were—in order of popularity—"passion," "love," "desire," "intimacy," "romance," and "lust." Based on these descriptors, it
should be clear that the fantasies we're talking about here all
involve some pretty intense feelings. There are obviously some
important differences in the nature of these feelings; however,
they can be grouped fairly easily into two distinct camps.

First, people who described their favorite fantasies in terms
of passion, desire, and lust tended to be looking for just one
thing: intense sexual attraction. Beyond that, the connection between the partners didn't necessarily go any deeper. In some
cases, my participants described a strong attraction that was
mutual, meaning the partners couldn't keep their hands off of
each other; however, most of them described an attraction that
flowed more in one direction than the other. Most commonly,
this involved fantasies about being sexually irresistible, such as
this straight woman in her twenties who said: "I love imagining
myself with a man who is crazy about my body, especially my
breasts. I love that feeling when I imagine that I am his fantasy
girl and my body is his fantasy body." Another woman, also in
her twenties but who identified herself as "mostly straight," described a similar desire to have a male partner who is totally
mad for her: "I guess it's just that my partner comes home and
wants me so bad that he throws me against a wall, rips off all

my clothes and fucks me right there in the living room. Not super kinky or weird, but it's nice to be wanted that much, you know?" Women aren't the only ones who fantasize about being wanted, though—a lot of men do, too, such as this straight man in his thirties whose ultimate fantasy is "to be wanted and desired over everything and everyone. For me, the technicalities don't matter. I only fantasize about my partner (or crush if I don't have one)." His point that the "technicalities don't matter" is emblematic of this type of fantasy: the specific sex acts themselves are secondary; what matters more than anything else is the intensity of passion and attraction.

By contrast, people who described their favorite fantasies in terms of love, intimacy, and romance tended to be looking for strong sexual attraction coupled with an intimate emotional connection—something along the lines of the epic love scenes you may have observed in films like *Ghost*, *Titanic*, or *The Notebook*. In other words, these fantasies tend to involve very passionate sex that is either an expression of the partners' deeper underlying feelings or a way of strengthening—or creating—an emotional bond. As you'll see below, these fantasies tended to be much more detailed than the passion-only fantasies, with participants taking a lot of time to set the scene. For example, one straight woman in her twenties described a very elaborate romance fantasy that begins on the beach: "I fantasize about making love to my partner in an intimate and romantic setting surrounded by the beach, listening to the sounds of the waves as I'm in his arms. He will caress me intensely, pulling my body close as we make love to the sounds of the ocean from morning until sunset. We will engage in multiple positions and in multiple sections of the house, with wet, soaked bodies entangled amongst one another. With passion, connection, and endless love." These fantasies aren't just about feeling connected to a current partner, though—sometimes they're about reconnecting with "the one who got away." For example, a "mostly straight" guy in his late teens said his favorite fantasy ends with him getting back together with his ex-girlfriend:

> My favorite fantasy is one in which I am back together with my ex, whom I care about very much. We would be making out in bed and I would slowly strip her clothes off. She would let me kiss my way down her body before pleasing her orally.... She would then mount me and we would make love for a while. In the throes of passion, she would leave long scratches down my back and maybe a few bite marks on my neck and shoulders. I would stand up and support her weight against the wall as her legs wrap around my waist and we continue in this position. Afterwards, we would transition to the bed and she would let me take her doggy style. Leaning over her, I would kiss her neck as I pump in and out of her. After having her climax once or twice, I would be nearing my own orgasm. She would kneel beside the bed and let me finish on her face and breasts.... We would then spend the day in bed, having sex and making love in various positions all day long....I would cook her a romantic dinner.... We would eventually fall asleep together, spooning. In the end, we would know that the next morning, we would both wake up having the love of our life next to us.

Other times, these fantasies are about creating a sense of intimacy with a completely new partner or someone with whom there is no prior sexual or romantic history. For example, a straight woman in her thirties talked about her desire to emotionally connect with a good friend through sex: "I fantasize about a man that I have desired for over a year.... I am hoping once I am divorced, one day we can explore a physical relationship. The fantasies are always different, perhaps like a future encounter. In some, I fantasize about him being confident, demanding and passionate; other times sweet, gentle, unsure. Perhaps they reflect what I need from him at the time. I have also fantasized about trying new sexual experiences with him. But most often it is achieving an emotional connection with him during urgent, hot, erotic, passionate sex." And yet other times, these fantasies are about the emotional connection one hopes to feel during one's very first sexual experience. In other words, people often romanticize the thought of losing their virginity, such as this gay man in his twenties:

I like to imagine what my first time having sex will be like....
My partner and I are in bed together naked. We both initiate
foreplay by kissing each other... caressing, cuddling, and whis-
pering sweet, erotic things to each other. He then moves on top
of me and starts licking my nipples and kissing the rest of my
upper body as he makes his way toward my private parts. He
then proceeds to give me fellatio. Sometimes I give my partner
fellatio too. My partner then proceeds to give me anal sex and
he gently thrusts into me while we hug and kiss each other.
We both climax together and we simply finish by lying together,
cuddling and kissing each other.

When looking at my participants' favorite fantasies of all time, passion and romance were nowhere near as popular as group sex, BDSM, and novelty. However, they turned out to be extraordinarily common when I looked at whether participants reported having *ever* had them. In fact, most of my participants—male and female—reported having previously fantasized about loved ones (current and former partners), about fulfilling a wide range of emotional needs (such as feeling loved, desired, and reassured), and about having sex in romantic settings. So, while these things don't tend to appear high on the list of people's favorite fantasies, it's clear that they do exist in almost everyone's fantasy repertoire. What this means is that most Americans don't just fancy an endless stream of mechanical sex acts—we also want to have sexual experiences that make us *feel* something. At least sometimes.

7. Homoeroticism and Gender-Bending

The final major fantasy theme I identified involves the desire for flexibility with respect to one's gender and/or sexuality. In other words, we're talking about fantasies in which people fundamentally reject binary notions of gender—that everyone is either male or female—and/or rigid notions of sexual orientation—for example, that being heterosexual means you can *only* be interested in partners of the opposite sex. In these fantasies, people are basically "bending" their gender or sexual orientation, such as by literally transforming into someone of a different gender, having a transsexual partner, or being heterosexual and desiring a same-sex experience.

This fantasy theme overlaps, to some extent, with both the novelty and taboo categories because it involves interjecting something new, exciting, and different into sex while simultaneously breaking cultural norms and rules for what people of a certain gender or sexual orientation are "supposed" to desire sexually. However, I thought it was important to cover these fantasies separately from the others because they suggest something far more important about Americans' sexual psychology than the fact that we're turned on by doing new and naughty things. These fantasies are revealing of an underlying sense of flexibility and fluidity in how Americans think about their gender and sexual identities.

There are really two broad categories of fantasies here. First, we have what I term *gender-bending* fantasies, in which a person may imagine cross-dressing or changing genders, or having sex with a cross-dressing or transgender partner. Second, we have what I term *sexual flexibility* fantasies, which feature sexual desires that are seemingly inconsistent with one's own sexual orientation. To give you a better flavor of what each of these fantasies is all about, we'll consider them separately below.

"Girls Who Are Boys Who Like Boys to Be Girls Who Do Boys Like They're Girls..."

If we look at the participants whose favorite fantasy of all time was gender-bending, the most common words used to describe their desires were "cross-dressing," "feminization," "genderplay," and "transgender/transsexual." Although these words obviously have very different meanings, I see them as really reflecting just two things. On the one hand, you have those folks whose interest in gender-bending involves getting it on after changing their own gender identity or role in some way. For example, some participants expressed an interest in cross-dressing. These folks reported that donning the garb of the other sex—or being forced to do so—is a sexually arousing act, like this straight guy in his twenties who told me that his biggest fantasy is simply to have sex in women's clothing: "I would like to have sex with a girl while I am dressed in women's clothes (like a dress, nightgown, bra and panties, etc.)." A man in his thirties who identified as "mostly straight" went a bit further in his fantasy, wanting to be feminized from head to toe: "I want to be feminized by my partner. I want her to turn me into a girl by dressing me in girls' clothes, keeping my body shaved, making me wear make-up. I want to be subservient to her, with her in control of whether or not I can have sexual release." As the latter example illustrates, there's sometimes an element of dominance-submission and/or humiliation involved in cross-dressing fantasies; however, in cases like this, it is almost exclusively men who want to be "feminized" by a dominant female partner—I didn't read a single fantasy about a woman who wanted to be masculinized by a male partner. Thus, at least for men, fantasies about cross-dressing may sometimes be viewed as an extension of a more general interest in BDSM.

That said, other folks' gender-bending fantasies went well beyond cross-dressing and involved a desire to *physically become* a member of the opposite sex, or to at least have the genitalia of the other sex. In other words, we're talking about fantasies that involve people transforming their sexual anatomy. The imagined transition can be grounded in reality, such as by undergoing genital surgery, or it can be a work of science fiction, like waking up in someone else's body (just as happened in the films *All of Me* and *The Hot Chick*). The arousal in these fantasies is often based on how transforming into the other sex makes them feel. For example, a woman who fantasizes about being a man may enjoy the feelings of dominance and power that go along with switching to a new gender identity, such as this "mostly straight" woman in her twenties described:

Since I was quite young I have used the fantasy of being a male and having a woman (usually myself to avoid feelings of guilt) give me a blow job. I enjoy this because imagining being a male puts me in a more dominant headspace, a selfish one, and I feel strongly desired since I know how confronting giving a blow job can be. I recently purchased a cock that I can wear and use as a double ended dildo which has allowed me to explore this fantasy further and I hope to one day find a partner that enjoys that role play with me.

Other times, however, the arousal may stem from an attraction to the opposite sex that is essentially turned inward, such as when a heterosexual man is aroused by the prospect of having a woman's body, like this "mostly straight" guy in his twenties: "I am a male but have autogynephilia; the attraction to thinking of myself as a woman. Although I have never crossdressed and do not desire to ever do so, I experience some of the most intense sexual desire when I imagine myself as a female. This is often imagined in a sexual capacity with one or more female partners.... Rarely does the desire to have sex with a fellow male come up, but will occasionally during these fantasies." I'm sure most of you aren't familiar with autogynephilia, a term that literally means "love of oneself as a woman," but some sex researchers have argued that this is what motivates a subset of biological men who seek gender affirmation surgery (formerly known as *sex reassignment surgery*).[15] We'll explore this concept in more detail later in the book, including some of the controversies surrounding it. However, for now, I just want to make the point that the fantasies I received about transsexualism paint a different picture than the narrative we've heard in the media, which suggests that transsexualism is only about "women trapped in men's bodies" and "men trapped in women's bodies"—a narrative suggesting that transitioning from one sex to the other is about *only* matters of identity, not sexuality. This is all we've ever heard reported when celebrities, like Caitlyn Jenner, publicly announce that they're changing genders. While I believe this media narrative is true in most cases, my survey results support the idea that, at least sometimes, transsexualism may be driven by sexual arousal at the thought of changing into the other sex.

Now, let's talk about the other class of gender-bending fantasies. Rather than bending one's own gender, these fantasies involve having sex with a partner who is bending *their* gender role or expression in some way. For example, this can mean having sex with someone who is cross-dressing, or who is being forced to cross-dress, as this "mostly straight" woman in her thirties described: "I dominate my male lover, make him wear lingerie. I have sex with my other male lover, who is young and fit and beautiful. I also make my lingerie-clad lover have sex with him." As you can see, when women fantasize about having sex with a cross-dressing male partner, there is sometimes an element of BDSM to it, just as we discussed in the case of men who fantasize about being cross-dressers.

Beyond desires for cross-dressing partners, some folks fantasize about having sex with persons who are transgender or transsexual, or who have both male and female genitalia. Of those participants who fantasized about this, the key thing that most people seemed to find arousing was the juxtaposition of masculine and feminine body features. For instance, one bisexual woman in her thirties described her desire to have sex with a partner who is biologically male below the waist but female above: "My ultimate fantasy would be to have sex with a transgender pre-op male. I love the look and feel of a woman-on-woman encounter. And I enjoy the penetration of a man. The visual of a female and the feeling of a man is a big turn on for me." A straight man in his fifties described his desire for a partner with a similar body:

I meet an attractive lady with long hair, nice round ass, sultry looking. She and I immediately desire each other and then she says she's different. She mentions she has a cock and that doesn't bother me. I lean over and we kiss passionately. We go up to a hotel room and she undresses, nice satin panties and beautiful tits. I rub her panties and feel her get erect. Pulling out her cock I stroke it and she moans. Laying on her back I keep stroking and then she takes over jerking off until a huge load shoots on her belly. She turns over and offers me her plump ass, I stroke myself erect and enter her, it's tight and firm, she starts stroking her cock again while I fuck her. I feel her starting to cum again and she tightens around my cock. After she cums again I pull out and I start stroking my cock, she fingers my ass and I explode all over her.

By contrast, a gay man in his twenties told me about his desire for a partner who had the reverse physical appearance—biologically female below the waist but male above: "Missionary position with a FTM [female-to-male] transgender person in which he fully resembled a man but had the female genitalia. This is the most recent and most intense fantasy that I can remember. I am a gay male and this is not a fantasy I thought I would ever have." All of these fantasies are examples of what have been dubbed *erotical illusions*, cases in which sexual cues are combined in a unique way that tricks the brain into feeling intense sexual arousal.[16] We'll return to this idea a little later in the book.

So just how common are all of these gender-bending fantasies we've been talking about? When looking at my participants' favorite fantasies of all time, gender-bending was relatively low on the list; however, when I asked whether people had ever fantasized about it, it turned out that a surprisingly large number had. For instance, about one-quarter of men and women had fantasized about cross-dressing, and nearly a third had fantasized about trading bodies with someone of the other sex. In addition, about one in four men and one in six women had fantasized about sex with a cross-dresser, and even more (about one in three men and one in four women) had fantasized about sex with a transsexual partner. My findings revealed that virtually all gender-bending fantasies were more common among men than women, for reasons we'll explore in the next chapter.

Sexual Flexibility Fantasies

Let's now consider those participants whose favorite fantasy of all time was sexual flexibility, or sex acts that are seemingly inconsistent with one's sexual orientation. The most common words used to describe these fantasies included "lesbian," "gay," and "bisexual." Therefore, what we're primarily talking about here are fantasies in which people—usually heterosexual—are aroused by the thought of having sex with someone of the same sex. This includes heterosexual women who fantasize about having sex with other women, such as this woman in her thirties: "I am a heterosexual female but I enjoy fantasizing about lesbian sex most often. I picture women going down on me or vice versa." A straight woman in her twenties expressed similar sentiments, though hers was based on a past real-life experience: "To have lesbian sex with my best friend, or to have lesbian sex with an experienced partner, without having romantic feelings/relationships/affiliation afterwards. I want to feel what it would be like to have casual lesbian sex. I often picture sucking my best friend's nipples at a sleep over and making her wet and rubbing our pussies together. I have mutually masturbated one of my good friends and I would love to do that again without feeling awkward or shamed."

Of course, there were also straight men who had fantasized about what it would be like to have sex with other men. Interestingly, these fantasies most commonly took place in the context of a threesome that also involved a woman, such as this straight guy in his twenties who told me: "I'm a straight guy, but I really want to have sex with a man and a woman at the same time. I want to be with the man as well, touch him, and have sex with him." Same goes for this straight twentysomething dude:

I describe myself as straight. However, I've always wanted to participate in a bisexual threesome with another man and a woman.... My fantasy does include giving and receiving oral sex to/from both the male and female participants. Also, me being between the male and female on my hands and knees going down on the female while the male is giving me anal. I would also enjoy giving the male anal. I would also like to be having vaginal intercourse with the woman while I'm getting it in the ass.... I would also like to be the male giving it to the other male in the above situations. It would be important for the woman involved to enjoy what was taking place between myself and the other man, as that's a huge turn-on for me.

It's interesting to note that, in both of these men's fantasies, the guys were quick to first establish their heterosexuality before declaring a desire to experiment sexually with men—but they really only wanted to do this experimenting in the presence of a woman. Why? Perhaps because it somehow feels less gay to have sex with a man when you're also having sex with a woman. In other words, maybe this scenario is less of a threat to these men in terms of how they view their own sexuality and/or sense of masculinity.

Although homoeroticism was the most common type of sexual flexibility fantasy, it's important to note that some people who identified as gay or lesbian said they had fantasies about heterosexual sex—in other words, lesbians who fantasized about sex with men and gay men who fantasized about sex with women. Case in point, a lesbian woman in her forties described her ultimate fantasy as "heterosexual sex. Male domination without violence. The male has to work hard to get the female to engage in sexual activity. Male is an alpha male with an athletic body. The female can't resist his sexual advances." Likewise, a man in his forties who identifies as "mostly gay" simply said "as a gay man, I often fantasize how it feels to penetrate a woman." As you can see, sexual flexibility is far from unique to heterosexuals—many gays and lesbians apparently find "heteroeroticism" appealing!

Sexual flexibility fantasies appear to be very common, especially among heterosexual women. In fact, 59 percent of the women I surveyed who identified as *exclusively* straight reported having had fantasies about sex with women! By contrast, just 26 percent of exclusively straight men I surveyed reported fantasies about sex with men. I should also say that lesbians were more likely to have heterosexual fantasies than were gay men, but overall, gays and lesbians were less likely to have heterosexual fantasies than straight folks were to have gay fantasies. Why is that? To some extent, these fantasies reflect basic curiosity about different kinds of sex, and gays and lesbians probably don't have as much curiosity about heterosexual sex as straight persons have about gay sex. The reason for this is that so many gays and lesbians have heterosexual experiences before coming out. In other words, the curiosity factor is likely to be lower for gays and lesbians because many of them have already experimented with heterosexual sex.

One other point I'd like to make here is that, while women had more fantasies about bending their sexual orientation than did men, men had more fantasies about bending their gender than did women. There are some fascinating psychological theories that can help to explain this gender difference, which we'll explore shortly.

The American Id, Revisited

By now, I hope your view of what's "normal" when it comes to sexual desire has expanded dramatically. Drawing from the findings of the largest survey of sexual fantasies in America,

I've shown that there are three things that almost everyone fantasizes about—group sex, BDSM, and novelty/adventure—and another four that many, if not most Americans get off on, too—taboo and forbidden activities, having a nonmonogamous relationship, passion and romance, and gender-bending and sexual flexibility.

Again, to be perfectly clear, I'm calling these fantasies "normal" in the sense that they are common. This is not to say that everyone who has one of these fantasies should go out and act on it—that's another matter entirely. For one thing, there are potential risks inherent in acting on any type of sexual fantasy that are important to consider—risks to both you and any relationship(s) you might have. For another, while perfectly normal to imagine, some of these fantasies would be illegal to act out (like voyeurism and sex in public) and/or have the potential to cause harm to others. Thus, we don't just want to start gratifying our ids no matter what they're telling us—but at the same time, we don't want to overcensor our ids, either, because that's a recipe for sexual dissatisfaction and frustration. We therefore need a delicate balancing act between the two, and how to accomplish that is something we'll come back to toward the end of the book.

3

Mars and Venus

How Do Men's and Women's Sexual Fantasies Differ?

John Gray's *Men Are from Mars, Women Are from Venus* is one of the best-selling books of all time. Its central premise—that men and women are so dramatically different in their psychology that we might as well think of them as coming from different planets—resonated with the American public in the 1990s. They purchased the book in droves, just as they did for Gray's follow-up sex manual (*Mars and Venus in the Bedroom*), which argued that, when it comes to sex, men and women have completely different physical and emotional needs. There's just one problem with both of these books: they're based on stereotypes, not science.

Men and women are not polar opposites when it comes to their sexual psychology. As you'll see in this chapter, most of the things that men fantasize about, women fantasize about as well—and vice versa. For example, gender stereotypes suggest that threesomes and group sex are typical fantasy themes for men but not women. These stereotypes also suggest that romance is a typical female but not male fantasy. However, the truth of the matter—and what my survey results reveal—is that most men and women have had both types of fantasies before. This tells us that there's actually a lot of commonality in what people desire when it comes to sex, regardless of their gender identity.

However, it's not fair to say that we're exactly the same, either. It's definitely not the case that men and women are identical with respect to what they fantasize about the most or how often they do it. For instance, although most men and women have had group-sex fantasies, men are more likely to have them, and they have them more often. Likewise, although most men and women have had passion and romance fantasies, these fantasies are more common among women, and women have them with greater frequency. These differences are nowhere near *Mars and Venus* proportions, but they still tell us something important about our sexual psychology. Therefore, we would be wise to take a close look at them.

Before we do, though, let's first dispense with the idea that the existence of a gender difference implies that one gender is somehow better than or inferior to another. Speaking about gender differences in any capacity has become increasingly controversial. In fact, I know a lot of scientists who won't speak publicly about *any* gender differences at all out of fear of backlash! That's problematic. Scientists shouldn't be afraid to talk about their data, and the public shouldn't be so quick to bash scientists who publish research that reveals politically inconvenient or uncomfortable truths. We need to be willing to consider data that challenge our worldview instead of burying our heads in the sand or just picking and choosing which scientific studies we're going to believe and which ones we're going to ignore. To the extent that we simply dismiss every study that challenges our beliefs as "fake news," we'll never truly understand how the world works. We'll also miss out on countless opportunities to apply science in ways that can better our lives.

The problem with discussing gender differences isn't really that we are afraid of finding out that men and women might be different—it's that we've been conditioned for far too long to believe that stereotypically feminine interests and desires are inferior and stereotypically masculine interests and desires are superior. That's the kind of thinking that's dangerous and that we should be standing against, not the very idea that gender differences themselves represent problems. As we go forward in this chapter, try to keep an open mind and remember that *difference* isn't a dirty word.

A Quick Sexual Vocabulary Lesson

Before we start exploring gender differences in sexual fantasy, it's important to step back and define a couple of key words and concepts. This will help you to better appreciate what some of the differences mean and where they might come from. In particular, it's essential that you understand the meaning of the terms *sexual orientation* and *sexual flexibility*. First, sexual orientation is something inborn that "orients" us toward a certain sex—usually toward women if you're male, and usually toward men if you're female. There's an abundance of genetic and neuroscience research suggesting that sexual orientation is influenced by biological factors early in life, especially the type and amount of sex hormones we're exposed to in utero.[1]

These hormones affect the development of the brain in numerous ways and ultimately lead to several important differences in brain structure and function between people who are attracted to the same sex and those attracted to the opposite sex.

Now, this isn't to suggest that prenatal hormonal exposure can only lead to two outcomes: a "gay brain" or a "straight brain." Biology is never so simple and predictable. Not only are we all exposed to different levels of hormones during fetal development for multiple reasons—including but not limited to variations in our mother's stress level, medication use, diet, and environment—but we also vary in our individual sensitivity to those hormones. As a result, our brains—and our sexualities—end up falling along a spectrum rather than existing as two discrete classes. The analogy I like to use is that we have two dials in the brain, one that controls attraction to men and one that controls attraction to women. In some cases, hormonal exposure turns one of these dials way up, resulting in a very strong orientation toward a particular sex. And if that dial is turned all the way up, perhaps it prevents the other dial from moving at all. In other cases, though, both dials might be turned to different degrees, with the end result being some variant of bisexuality. And in yet other cases, neither dial moves at all, resulting in a total lack of sexual attraction, or asexuality.

In short, sexual orientation is the degree to which we are biologically predisposed to desiring men, women, both, or neither. In order to facilitate reproduction and the survival of our species, though, most people wind up with a moderate to strong orientation toward the opposite sex—an orientation that emerges around puberty and remains relatively stable throughout one's life.

By contrast, sexual flexibility is a totally separate aspect of the sexual brain that operates alongside our sexual orientation. To go back to my earlier analogy, think of sexual flexibility as a third dial that can be turned completely, partially, or not at all. Sexual flexibility is a willingness to deviate not only from our sexual orientation but also from what our culture and society have told us we should want when it comes to sex. In other words, it's our degree of comfort with trying new things and bucking sexual norms. We all have some degree of sexual flexibility—it's just that some folks only have a little, while others have a lot. For those who are low on flexibility, their sexual orientation will appear pretty stable over the life span, barring some extraordinary circumstances. For instance, consider a man with a strong heterosexual orientation who is low on sexual flexibility (in other words, his flexibility dial is just slightly turned up)—he might ultimately have sex with other men, but only if his access to female partners is severely limited, such as if he is in an all-male prison, attending an all-male boarding school, or stranded on a desert island where there are no women around. If his testosterone levels are high enough, he's feeling horny, and he is unable to obtain partners of the sex he's oriented toward, he may pursue same-sex contact—but, again, only in the most extraordinary of circumstances. Now, if we instead imagine that this same man has a high degree of sexual flexibility (that is, his dial is turned up as high as it goes), he might not need such extreme circumstances to pursue same-sex contact. For instance, if his female partner really wants to have a threesome with another man, he might readily oblige. Or if he is single and finds himself the object of affection of a gay man he meets at a party, he might agree to receive a blow job after having a drink or two. However, it's important to note that he'd still wake up heterosexual the next morning in both cases, because his strong underlying orientation toward women would not have changed. (Remember, orientation is controlled by totally different dials.)

Your degree of sexual flexibility therefore says a lot about who you're willing to have sex with and under what circumstances. However, sexual flexibility is also, to some extent, a general willingness to try to new sexual things—especially things that might be socially or culturally forbidden. This idea—that sexual flexibility isn't limited to the gender of your partner—is not something that many other scientists have previously argued, but it's something that's strongly supported by my survey data. When I looked at participants who said that they were either exclusively gay or straight, I found that those who had fantasies about same-sex contact were more likely to have a whole host of other sexual fantasies that deviate from what many people consider "normal." For instance, they were more likely to fantasize about being with partners of different races, engaging in BDSM sex, having group sex, and being consensually nonmonogamous, among other things. In other words, we're talking about a very general erotic flexibility here that goes well beyond being flexible about the gender of one's partner. It includes flexibility with respect to other partner characteristics, such as race, as well as flexibility in terms of trying new sex acts, such as BDSM.

Got it? Good. With these definitions in mind, think back to when we talked about homoeroticism fantasies. If you'll recall, I found that nearly two-thirds of women who said they were exclusively heterosexual had same-sex fantasies; by contrast, the number of exclusively straight men who had same-sex fantasies was less than half that. This tells us that women's fantasy partners are less likely to match up with their sexual orientation compared to men. Why is that? As I'll explain below, scientists believe it's because women's sexual flexibility dials tend to be turned up higher than men's.

No, Not All Women Are Bisexual—but Women Do Have a More Flexible Sexuality

A lot of Americans are under the impression that all women are secretly bisexual—men, not so much. In fact, a lot of people question whether male bisexuality is even a thing. This kind of thinking reminds me of scene from the classic television series *Sex and the City* in which Carrie Bradshaw famously mused, "I did the 'date a bisexual guy' thing in college, but in the end they all ended up with men. . . . I'm not even sure bisexuality exists. I think it's just a layover on the way to gaytown."[2]

The truth of the matter is that both of these beliefs about bisexuality—that all women are bi and all men are either straight or gay—are incorrect. Men can indeed be bisexual. And while women are more likely than men to be bisexual, it's far from the case that *all* women are. The reason we perceive bisexuality as being so common among women isn't necessarily that women are more likely to have both of their sexual orientation dials turned up. It's that their third dial, the one that gives them their sexual flexibility, is usually turned up a little higher than men's. There is a large and growing body of research supporting this idea.

Much of the research in this area has focused on how our genitals respond when we're shown different types of pornography.[3]

The way these studies usually go is that men and women are first hooked up to devices that record changes in blood flow to the genitals. Specifically, men are given a circular ring to put around the penis that records changes in erection size, whereas women are given a tampon-shaped device to insert in the vagina that measures blood flow to the vaginal area by emitting light and recording how much is reflected back via a photocell. Basically, as more blood flows to the vaginal tissues, more light is reflected back, and that is registered as increased arousal. Once these devices are in place, participants watch a series of brief porn videos in a random order, usually separated by some nonarousing nature videos.

The typical pattern that emerges is that straight men show the strongest arousal to lesbian porn. Of course, they show significant arousal to heterosexual porn, too; however, they show relatively little arousal when watching gay male porn. (Except for the really homophobic "straight" men—it turns out that a lot of them are actually turned on by videos of dudes getting it on. In other words, some homophobes doth protest too much.[4]) Likewise, gay men show the strongest arousal in response to gay porn. They show significant arousal in response to heterosexual porn as well, but—not surprisingly—lesbian porn doesn't do much for gay guys.

By contrast, women—especially heterosexual-identifying women—tend to show substantial genital arousal in response to all kinds of porn, regardless of the gender of the actors in the videos. This pattern suggests that women's arousal is fairly flexible, whereas men's seems to be more fixed with respect to their partners' gender.

As further support for this idea that women have a more flexible sexuality, study after study has found that women's sexual behavior is more variable than men's over the course of their lives. For example, in his review of more than forty years of research on differences in male and female sexual behavior, social psychologist Roy Baumeister discovered that—among other things—women are more likely to have a same-sex experience in prison than men, despite what the popular media might lead you to believe (*Orange Is the New Black* notwithstanding).[5] Likewise, among people who are into swinging and group sex, he found that same-sex experiences are far more common among women than men.

So what does all of this mean? Why do women seem to be more flexible when it comes to the gender of their partners? Some have argued that there's a cultural explanation. Because male homosexuality has, at least in recent history, been more socially reviled than female homosexuality, perhaps men's sexual fantasies and desires are more inhibited with respect to partner gender. In other words, perhaps men have been the targets of greater cultural conditioning. However, one piece of evidence that argues against this point is that, when you look at genital arousal patterns of male-to-female transsexuals, their responses don't match up with those of women—instead, they look more like those of men in that they show far more arousal to one gender than the other.[6] In light of this, some have suggested that the underlying reason might be biological or evolutionary instead of cultural.

One evolutionary hypothesis is that it was adaptive for women to evolve a flexible sexuality because this would have assisted our female ancestors in cases where their male partners abandoned them or were killed.[7] Think about it this way: thousands of years ago, it would have been difficult for women to survive alone if they were pregnant or had children by a man who was no longer in the picture (e.g., if the guy died or went to shack up with someone else). Finding a man who would be willing to make the sacrifices necessary to raise another man's children would have been challenging; hence, some scientists have argued that it would have improved women's (and their children's) odds of survival if women could reorient their attraction to other women, effectively doubling their potential pool of alternatives for partnering up and sharing responsibilities.

Another evolutionary hypothesis is that perhaps women's greater sexual flexibility evolved in response to men's greater social power.[8] The basic idea is that, throughout most of recorded history, men have held more power over women economically and politically. They've also typically held more physical power due to sex differences in strength and size. According to this reasoning, perhaps women became more erotically flexible in order to reduce the risk of harm being inflicted upon them during sexual disputes with men. Put another way, holding lesser power for so many millennia may have led women to become more sexually flexible in the interest of survival and self-preservation.

Yet one other possibility is that perhaps men and women have different sexual imprinting windows, periods of time during which one can learn new sexual interests. Some scientists believe that men undergo a very brief sexual imprinting period during adolescence and that, once the imprinting window closes, it becomes harder for them to develop new sexual interests. Another way to think of this is that maybe men tend to experience something that dials down their sexual flexibility at a young age. For instance, perhaps the hormonal surges boys experience during adolescence have the potential to turn their flexibility dials back a bit, or maybe turn them off completely in some cases. The appeal of this theory is that it helps to explain why so many men with fetishes can trace them back to a very early sexual experience, such as trying on their mother's shoes or fooling around with the family pet. Another advantage of this theory is that it can help to explain why men are more likely to engage in bisexual behavior during adolescence than at any other time in their lives. Many are skeptical of this theory, though, because the evidence is based almost entirely on retrospective recall of previous sexual behaviors. Maybe it's just easier to recall early sexual experiences that are consistent with our current interests and desires because those experiences are more salient in our memories. This raises the question of whether early sexual experiences shape our desires or whether our desires shape what we remember of our early sexual experiences and how we label and interpret them. Of course, maybe there's a bit of both going on.

We can't say for sure which, if any, of these explanations is correct, or whether there's potentially some truth to all of them. However, what's clear is that there are multiple theories—both cultural and evolutionary—that could potentially account for the consistent observation that women seem to have greater sexual flexibility than men. These theories help to explain my survey results showing that women, particularly those who are heterosexual, are more malleable with respect to the gender of their fantasy partners than men. However, they also help to explain a number of the other gender differences in fantasy content that emerged in my survey. Below, we'll take a look at some of the other differences that I discovered and consider how women's greater sexual flexibility might explain them; of course, as you'll see, this isn't the only way to explain all of these gender differences. In fact, some of the gender differences we'll explore might be due to factors that have little—perhaps nothing—to do with sexual flexibility.

Women Care Less About Who Their Partners Are but More About Where They Have Sex

I asked my participants to rate how arousing they found each of the following aspects of their favorite sexual fantasy of all time: the specific sex act that took place, the person(s) they had sex with, and where they did it. I then compared men's and women's answers. What I found was that there were no overall gender differences when it came to how they felt about what they did. That is, men and women rated the sex act itself as equally important in their fantasies. The who and where questions were a whole other story, though.

On average, men reported more arousal from who their fantasy partners were than women did. I drilled down into specific kinds of fantasies to see whether this pattern was consistent, and it was—in every type of fantasy in which there was a gender difference, it was always men who were more aroused by whom they were having sex with. Why is that? Well, the idea that women have greater sexual flexibility than men provides one compelling explanation. If women's sexuality is simply more flexible by nature, then it makes sense that, when it comes to their sexual fantasies, the details of the person(s) they're having sex with shouldn't be quite as important.

There's at least one other way of explaining this finding, though, and after reading through the thousands of fantasies I collected, it seems pretty plausible, too (it's also consistent with previously published research on sexual fantasy): women appear more likely than men to see themselves as the object of desire in their sexual fantasies.[9] Therefore, having a specific person in mind may not matter as much to women because they themselves are usually—though certainly not always—the focus of the fantasy, not their partners. By contrast, it appears that men are more likely than women to view their fantasy selves not as objects of desire but as acting on an object of desire, which would make having a specific partner in mind more important for men.

With that said, it's worth noting that there are certain kinds of fantasies where men and women care equally about who their partners are. For example, when looking at passion and romance fantasies, no gender difference emerged when it came to the importance placed on the partner. This makes sense, given that feelings of romance and passion are usually tied to a specific person—those aren't emotions we usually feel for completely random or anonymous people.

When it came to where their fantasies took place, women cared more about the setting than men. And, again, when looking at specific types of fantasies, the direction of the gender difference was consistent every time it emerged. So why does the setting matter more to women than to men, especially if women have a more flexible sexuality? I suspect it has something to do with another gender difference we'll explore later in this chapter, which is that women are more likely to have emotion-based fantasies than men. Having a specific setting in mind may be important for creating a certain tone or mood that helps to ensure a particular emotional need is met. Consistent with this reasoning, I found that the more importance participants placed on the setting, the more likely they were to have fantasies about meeting emotional needs. To be clear, this is not to say that the setting always matters more to women than men. For instance, in the case of group sex, BDSM, and romance fantasies, men and women rated the setting as equally important (or, to be more precise, unimportant). This is likely because the key elements of those fantasies are the sexual activities and/or people—not where the sex takes place. In other words, while women may derive more arousal from fantasy settings on average, women don't always place more importance on the location than men.

"There's a Certain Satisfaction in a Little Bit of Pain": Why Women Have More BDSM Fantasies Than Men

When the first film adaptation of the popular BDSM-themed novel *Fifty Shades of Grey* landed in movie theaters, the audience largely consisted of women—in fact, they made up more than two-thirds of ticket buyers on opening weekend![10] What accounts for this? My survey results offer some insight: women have more BDSM fantasies of almost every type than men. Therefore, it only makes sense that a phenomenon like *Fifty Shades* wouldn't have equally strong appeal for both sexes.

So why do women fantasize about almost all of these forms of kinky sex more than men? This is another difference that can potentially be explained by women's greater sexual flexibility. Recall that sexual flexibility isn't just about being flexible with respect to who your partner is—it also includes flexibility with respect to sexual activities. However, that's not the only possible explanation. It could also be that women's greater interest in BDSM might have something to do with the idea that women are more likely than men to fantasize about being the object of desire. For example, if you think about something like bondage, well, being tied up is the epitome of becoming a sex object, especially when you think back to some of the sample bondage fantasies we considered earlier in this book. This same reasoning could help to explain why women also have more discipline, submission, and masochism fantasies, because unquestioningly following orders, submitting to others, and receiving pain are all experiences that depersonalize us to some extent—they transform us from persons to objects. This same transformation does not occur in dominance scenarios, though, which was the one kind of BDSM fantasy that women had less of than men. So the overall pattern here makes sense.

The one survey result this women-as-objects-of-desire line of reasoning doesn't quite explain is the fact that women actually reported more frequent sadism fantasies—that is, fantasies about giving pain—than men. This finding was quite surprising to me. Whereas sadism has long been thought to be an almost exclusively male sexual interest, my survey results suggest that women are actually a little more into it than men—at least with respect to the types of sadistic activities I inquired about, which focused on things like spanking, biting, and dripping hot wax on a partner. It's possible the results might have been different had I had focused on more intense ways of inflicting pain, like whipping. While we can't rule out this possibility, it's important to note that the gender difference I observed in sadism fantasies was quite small and nowhere near as large as what I saw in the other areas of BDSM. For instance, women were twice as likely as men to say that they often have bondage fantasies and almost four times as likely to say they often fantasize about masochism. By contrast, women were just 17 percent more likely to report frequent sadism fantasies. It's also important to note that, while most men and women had fantasized about sadism before, this element of BDSM was the one they both fantasized about least often. In other words, we're dealing with a very small difference in a relatively low-frequency fantasy. Therefore, we should be cautious about overinterpreting it, especially given that this finding isn't perfectly consistent with past research.

There's at least one other theory that can help to explain why women find most kinds of BDSM more arousing than men, which is the idea that BDSM experiences offer an escape from self-awareness.[11] With masochism fantasies in particular, the physical sensations of pain can help to take you out of your head, thereby distracting you from any sexual hang-ups and anxieties that might otherwise diminish arousal. Given that women are more likely than men to receive cultural messages that they're not supposed to like or want sex, sexual activities like BDSM that help to distract women from culturally induced sexual anxiety might be particularly appealing to them.

Why Women Have More Emotion-Based Fantasies Than Men

I asked my survey participants how often they had fantasies about meeting a wide range of emotional needs. These included receiving approval, feeling loved or appreciated, feeling sexually desired, being sexually irresistible, feeling reassured, feeling sexually competent, and emotionally connecting with a partner. Women reported having every single one of these emotion-based fantasies more often than men. However, this isn't to say that men don't have emotion-based fantasies at all or that they only have them on rare occasions—far from it! In fact, the majority of men I surveyed said they fantasized about meeting all of these emotional needs at least sometimes. For both men and women, feeling desired, sexually competent, and irresistible were the most common emotional needs they fantasized about meeting.

I should also say that both men *and* women were far more likely to fantasize about meeting emotional needs than they were to fantasize about emotionless sex. In fact, the vast majority of both men and women (more than 70 percent) said that they rarely or never have fantasies about emotionless sex. This tells us that our fantasies are more likely than not to have an emotional element to them, regardless of our gender. It also challenges gender stereotypes about the role of emotion in sexual fantasy. While women certainly have more emotional content in their fantasies than men on average, there's still a heck of a lot of emotion in men's sexual fantasies.

So why do women have more emotion-based fantasies? This is one case where women's greater sexual flexibility doesn't offer a compelling rationale. In fact, when I looked at my data, being more flexible with respect to the gender of one's partner was not linked to having more fantasies about meeting emotional needs—just the opposite! Among exclusively heterosexual women, the more same-sex fantasies they had, the fewer emotion-based fantasies they reported. The same was true for exclusively straight men—more same-sex fantasies were linked to fewer emotion fantasies.

If sexual flexibility isn't the explanation, then what is? One possibility is that women's greater interest in emotion-based fantasies is learned. American women have long been the recipients of cultural messages that sex should be an inherently emotional experience for them and that they're not supposed to want casual, no-strings-attached sex. So it could be that women have just been conditioned to think about sex in more emotional terms. Along these same lines, it's also possible that fantasizing about emotional connection and fulfillment could be a way that some women relieve themselves of feelings of guilt or shame over sexual fantasies that involve culturally taboo activities. For instance, adding an emotional element to a casual-sex fantasy might lead to less guilt about desiring casual sex.

An alternative view is that perhaps women evolved to have emotion-based fantasies more often. Evolutionary psychologists argue that humans—like all other species—are motivated to pass their genes along to future generations; however, because reproduction is much more costly for women than it is for men, it makes sense that the sexes would have evolved different mating strategies that reflect the vastly different biological realities they face. For men, it would be adaptive to have greater ability to separate sex from emotion because this would increase their odds of pursuing mating opportunities with a wider range of partners, thereby enhancing their reproductive potential. For women, though, it would be adaptive to seek more connection between sex and emotion in the interest of promoting long-term relationships with men who are going to stick around and help care for any children they father. Thus, from the evolutionary viewpoint, it would make sense for women's fantasies to be somewhat more emotional and less casual in general than men's.

Up until this point, we've focused on the fantasy themes that are more common among women, including less emphasis on who their partner is (and their partner's gender), more emphasis on the setting, more interest in BDSM, and more emotional content. Now let's take a look at the fantasy themes that are more common among men.

Plays Well in Groups: Why Men Have More Group-Sex Fantasies Than Women

The men who took my survey fantasized about all forms of group sex—threesomes, gangbangs, and orgies—more often than women. Again, to be clear, group-sex fantasies are very popular among women, and most women have had them. It's just that men seem a bit more drawn to scenarios in which they're having sex with multiple partners at the same time.

So why is that? Evolutionary psychologists have argued that it has something to do with sperm competition. When men are in sexual situations in which multiple guys are having sex with the same women, their sperm are no longer just competing against each other to reach the egg first—they're competing against other men's swimmers, too. It is thought that men's brains and bodies evolved to take action in these situations in order to help them compete more effectively.

Consider this: in a study in which researchers collected straight men's ejaculate after they masturbated to one of two different pornos, they found that guys who viewed a gangbang scenario in which multiple men were having sex with the same woman released more active sperm than guys who watched a video of lesbian group sex.[12] In other words, it seems that men are unknowingly increasing the sperm level in their ejaculate in response to the specter of competition.

Scientists have also found that when heterosexual men suspect a female partner of having recently cheated, they engage in harder and faster thrusting the next time they have sex.[13] It seems that when men believe that another guy has had sex with their partner, they become more vigorous in bed. The thought is that these men are subconsciously trying to remove sperm that may have been deposited by male rivals—something researchers claim the human penis was designed by evolution to do. As some evidence for this idea, consider a study in which researchers took dildos of different shapes and sizes and stuffed them into artificial vaginas loaded with simulated semen. (By the way, should you need to make your own simulated semen, all you need to do is mix seven milliliters of room temperature water with 7.16 grams of cornstarch and stir for five minutes. As reported in a 2003 journal article, "this recipe was judged by three sexually experienced males to best approximate the viscosity and texture of human seminal fluid."[14]) The scientists found that the dildo that most closely approximated the shape of a real-life penis displaced the most simulated semen, particularly when it was thrust deeply. Put another way, men's penises aren't just vessels for depositing semen—they're also tools for removing semen left behind by other men. However, to be most effective at semen removal, guys need to be extra energetic in bed, so it would make sense that sperm competition scenarios would generate high levels of sexual arousal and excitement in men.

Although evidence for the sperm competition theory is growing, it remains a somewhat controversial topic, and more research is needed. However, to the extent that it's true, it offers a fascinating explanation for why men have more group-sex fantasies than women.

Deviant Desires: Why Men Have More Taboo Fantasies Than Women

Men were also more likely than women to fantasize about the vast majority of taboo acts I inquired about on my survey, including voyeurism, exhibitionism, incest, and fetishism. And when it came to the most deviant and extreme fantasies, like pedophilia and bug chasing (intentionally contracting an STD), men far outnumbered women. I wasn't surprised to find this because most research has shown that taboo sexual interests are largely, though certainly not exclusively, a male phenomenon.[15]

There were a couple of taboo fantasies I inquired about that men and women were equally likely to report having: sex with animals, being a furry (dressing up as an animal to have sex), frotteurism (rubbing up against an unsuspecting stranger in a public place), and necrophilia (sex with a corpse). This runs contrary to previous studies showing that men are primarily the ones who have these particular interests. However, those studies were typically based on very small samples of people who had actually acted out these behaviors in real life. To the extent that men are more likely to act on taboo fantasies than women (or are more likely to be caught acting on taboo fantasies), this could explain the discrepancy between my findings and other studies. Interestingly, there was just one taboo on my survey that women were substantially more likely to fantasize about than men, which was being an adult baby (dressing up, acting like, and/or being treated as an infant). However, this makes sense because adult baby fantasies often involve themes of masochism and submission, such as getting spanked. Therefore, these fantasies might just be an outgrowth of women's greater attraction to BDSM. With all of that said, my results suggest that women probably have more taboo sexual interests than we've been led to believe; overall, though, they don't have quite as many as men.

So why do men have more taboo sexual fantasies? I suspect that a big part of the reason for this is that men tend to have more sensation-seeking tendencies than women. Study after study (my survey included) has found this to be the case— that men have a higher threshold for excitement and are simply more willing to engage in intense activities, including both those that are sexual and nonsexual in nature.[16] Before we go on, note that sensation seeking (which men are higher in) is distinct from sexual flexibility (which women are higher in). Sexual flexibility simply refers to a general openness to trying new things and deviating from sexual norms. Being open to new experiences (i.e., being sexually flexible) isn't the same as preferring or needing intense experiences in order to get off. With that said, it would make sense that men would be more drawn to sexual taboos because violating them offers just the kind of stimulation and excitement that sensation seekers are looking for. So why are men more likely to be sensation seekers? Some argue that it's due to gender stereotypes and cultural factors shaping men's and women's personalities; however, others argue that we simply evolved this way. From an evolutionary perspective, if sensation seeking in general were to assist men when it came to obtaining resources or competing for mates, then nature would have selected for this trait in men. Likewise, if sensation seeking is detrimental to women due to their higher cost of reproduction, then women should have evolved to be more averse to risks of all sorts.

So sensation seeking might open the door to men's exploring more taboos in the first place; however, it's important to note that once men start exploring taboo interests, they tend to stick. This may be because, again, men's sexuality tends to be more fixed than women's, meaning that once men develop a sexual interest, they tend to maintain it.

On a side note, men's greater interest in sexual taboos might also have something to do with the fact that they're more likely than women to have compulsive sexual tendencies. Several studies—and my survey—have found that men tend to be higher on sexual compulsivity and, further, that greater compulsivity is linked to more taboo sexual desires.[17] By "compulsive tendencies," I mean sexual thoughts and behaviors that one struggles to manage—in other words, people with compulsive tendencies don't feel like they have control over their sexual desires. While we don't fully understand the reason(s) for this gender difference in sexual compulsivity, one thing we do know is that not everyone who feels their sexual urges are out of control truly has *compulsive* tendencies. I say this because research has found that people who feel morally conflicted about their sexual desires have a tendency to label those desires as being "out of control."[18] What this means is that the link between taboo interests and perceived sexual compulsivity sometimes reflects nothing more than moral qualms with one's fantasy content. Consistent with this idea, the men who took my survey reported feeling more guilt about their sexual fantasies on average than women. This finding probably strikes many as counterintuitive, given that we live in a world where women tend to be judged more harshly than men just for being desirous of sex. Nonetheless, what this tells us is that perhaps part of the reason many men with taboo desires report feeling as though they can't control their sexual urges is that men are simply more ashamed of their sexual desires than are women.

Why Men Have More Gender-Bending Fantasies Than Women

One final type of sexual fantasy where there was a major difference between men and women was in the area of gender-bending. Whereas women seem to be more flexible than men when it comes to experimenting with their sexual orientation, men seem to be more flexible than women when it comes to experimenting with their own and their partners' gender identities. Not only do men fantasize more often than women about having sex with partners who are cross-dressers or transsexuals, but they also fantasize more about bending their own gender through cross-dressing or physically changing their bodies. Something that may surprise you about both of these kinds of fantasies is that the men who are most likely to have them are heterosexual—not gay or bisexual.

Let's talk first about men who are into gender-bending partners. In psychological terms, these guys are known as *gynandromorphophiles* (how's that for a tongue twister?), which is basically an elaborate way of saying they're into sex partners who possess both male and female physical characteristics.

Again, to be clear, research finds that these guys mostly identify as heterosexual, and genital-arousal studies comparing gynandromorphophilic males to heterosexual and homosexual
men finds that their arousal patterns look more like straight
guys' than gay guys'.[19] In other words, they are more aroused
by images of women than they are by images of men—however,
more than anything else, they are aroused by photos and
videos of people who have both male and female physical
characteristics—people who are often referred to in the porn
world by the very non-PC term *she-male*.

The appeal of gynandromorphophilia is thought to stem from
what neuroscientists Ogi Ogas and Sai Gaddam have termed
erotical illusions: unique combinations of sexual cues that, together, produce an extremely intense state of sexual arousal—
far more than they would stimulate on their own.[20] In other
words, when you combine strong physical cues of both masculinity and femininity, the result can be a very powerful erotic
stimulus. But why would this affect men more than women? According to Ogas and Gaddam, it could be because men are more
erotically responsive to visual sexual cues than women, something that could also explain why men in general tend to watch
so much more porn. However, other scientists have questioned
this explanation, arguing that the idea of men being more vi-
sually aroused is a myth and that men's greater porn-watching
stems primarily from the fact that most porn is made by men,
for men.

Now, let's address the guys who fantasize about bending their
own gender. In psychological terms, they are known as *autogynephiles*, a term that refers to feeling sexual arousal in response
to the thought or image of oneself as a woman. Psychologist

Ray Blanchard has described four different types of autogynephilia, which vary in terms of the kinds of thoughts and/
or behaviors that are sexually arousing: (1) wearing women's
clothing (i.e., cross-dressing), (2) acting or behaving in a feminine manner, (3) fantasizing about having female bodily func-
tions, and (4) imagining having a woman's body or body parts.[21]
Autogynephilic men can be attracted to men, women, both, or
neither—it does not necessarily say anything about their sexual
orientation.

Many psychologists argue that autogynephilia is one type of
transsexualism. However, it is important to clarify that not all
male-to-female transsexuals are autogynephiles—thus, it is not
the case that every natal man who desires to become a woman
does so because he is sexually aroused by the thought of seeing
himself as such. Most transsexuals are probably best described
as being motivated not by sexual desire but by feeling trapped
in the body of the wrong sex. Also, given all of the varieties of
autogynephilia that have been described, it is not accurate to
say that all autogynephiles are transsexuals, either.

The origins of autogynephilia and why men are more likely
to be aroused by the thought of becoming the other sex are
not well understood. However, when you think about it, violating gender roles and expectations has historically been a
major social and cultural taboo, so perhaps this desire stems
from men's greater tendency to develop taboo sexual interests
more generally. As some support for this idea, I found that the
men who reported autogynephilia fantasies were more likely
to report having almost every other taboo fantasy I inquired
about. So whatever draws men to the taboo in the first place
may also draw them to autogynephilia. In addition, I found that

autogynephilia fantasies were related to reporting more compulsive sexual tendencies. Although this association was small, it is consistent with the idea that taboo interests may persist in some men because men are more likely to report compulsive sexual urges. Or maybe it just signifies that many men with autogynephilia fantasies feel morally conflicted about these desires, given that shame and guilt are linked more generally to labeling one's sexual desires as compulsive or beyond one's control.

One other interesting thing I discovered about autogynephilia fantasies is that they were related more generally to fantasies about becoming someone or something else entirely, such as being an adult baby or a furry. What do all three of these fantasies have in common? Well, they're all fundamentally about escaping one's sense of self. This suggests to me that men who are seeking an escape from self-awareness or reality might be predisposed to having not just autogynephilia fantasies but also a range of other fantasies about physical transformation.

You might be wondering whether there's a counterpart to autogynephilia among women, and there is—it's known as *autoandrophilia*, which refers to women who are sexually aroused by the thought or image of themselves as men. Far less is known about autoandrophilia than autogynephilia. In fact, Ray Blanchard, who did most of the pioneering research on autogynephilia, is on the record as recently as 2013 claiming, "I don't think the phenomenon even exists."[22] However, if the results of my fantasy survey are any indication, autoandrophilia most definitely is real, and it's probably more common than Blanchard thinks. Indeed, I found that 11 percent of the women I surveyed reported sexual fantasies about becoming men and that

20 percent had fantasized about dressing up as men (although I should clarify that just 2–3 percent said they fantasized about these things often, meaning autoandrophilia rarely becomes women's preferred fantasy content).

I would be remiss if I didn't stop for a moment and acknowledge that there's a lot of controversy surrounding the concept of autogynephilia. In fact, I know that just by writing about it I will invite some negative criticism and perhaps inspire some nasty book reviews. The critiques of this concept have been thoroughly addressed elsewhere and can be easily and freely accessed online, so I won't get into them here except to mention that many in the trans community are uncomfortable with the very concept of autogynephilia because they see it as pathologizing for transsexuals due to the fact that it suggests an underlying sexual motivation for some members of the trans community. Some are also concerned that acceptance of this theory will set back the fight for transgender rights. While I certainly understand and appreciate these concerns, I am not able to ignore the accumulated evidence, which suggests that there are different types of trans persons: some who are autogynephilic, some who are autoandrophilic, and some who are neither. Though I believe the vast majority of trans persons aren't autogynephilic or autoandrophilic, as a scientist, I think it's important that we recognize this diversity instead of pretending it doesn't exist just because we don't like the implications.

With that said, let me be clear that I personally support a social agenda of trans inclusiveness. I believe that *all* trans persons deserve our respect and acceptance—and those who have a desire to undergo a physical transition should be able to do so because the evidence is clear that it doesn't hurt; rather, it helps.[23] Moreover, I believe that trans persons deserve equal rights and should be able to live their lives as they please without be persecuted for doing so, regardless of whether they are autogynephilic, autoandrophilic, or neither. In short, I am a trans ally. However, I am also a scientist—and being a scientist means not letting my personal beliefs stand in the way of my ability to accept and report what the data say.

So What Have We Learned from All of This?

The conclusion I do *not* want you to take from this chapter is that, when it comes to sexual desire, men are from Mars and women are from Venus. We've certainly discussed a lot of ways that men's and women's sexual fantasies differ. We've also discussed how a lot of those differences may stem from fundamental underlying differences between female and male sexualities—most notably, the idea that women's sexuality is more flexible than men's. Attending to these differences is important because it can help us to better understand, for example, why men and women don't always agree on what they want when it comes to sex and why they may find different kinds of pornography to be sexually arousing. That said, the fantasy worlds that populate our minds are much more alike than they are different. Please keep in mind that the seven major fantasy themes discussed earlier characterize both male *and* female sexual desire. Most men and women are fantasizing about the same things; the main difference is really in the frequency with which they have a given type of fantasy.

4

What Do Your Sexual Fantasies Say About You?

The Fifteen Questions That Reveal Your Secret Sexual Desires

Tell me a little bit about you, and I'll tell you what your fantasies are.

Your answers to fifteen simple questions can help me to predict what types of things are likely to turn you on—and what types of things are likely to turn you off. All I need is a little information about your demographic background, your personality, and your sexual history. Below, we'll explore each of these fifteen questions in turn and explain why they're important for understanding Americans' sexual desires. I'll draw upon insights gleaned from my survey, but I'll also bring in the science that can help you to better understand what your fantasies say about who you are and where you are in life. Note that your gender, of course, also says a lot about your desires; however, because gender was considered extensively in the previous chapter, we won't really be talking about it much here.

Before we begin exploring the origins of our fantasies, let me first caution you that there isn't a singular cause for any of the fantasies mentioned in this book. What this means is that, although Americans share a lot of fantasies in common, they don't necessarily develop those fantasies for the same reasons. Thus, as we start exploring where our fantasies come from, please keep in mind that there are multiple routes to any given fantasy. Remember, too, that a fantasy can be constructed in many different ways depending on the person. So, while two people might have fantasies that reflect the same general theme—like BDSM—odds are that those fantasies will have very distinct scripts.

I should also say that if we discuss a particular trait you have that's linked to greater odds of having a certain fantasy, but you don't happen to have that fantasy, it doesn't necessarily mean that the data are wrong or that there's something wrong with you. Remember that our fantasies have complex origins. Your personality and life experiences don't make you destined to have certain fantasies—at most, they simply increase the likelihood that you'll fantasize about some things more than others. Whether we actually come to fantasize about a given person, place, or thing depends upon the convergence of several factors. Therefore, we really need to look at a person's entire constellation of traits to understand that individual's fantasies, as opposed to looking at just one trait in isolation.

It's worth mentioning that there are some personality traits and characteristics that are linked to fantasizing more about almost *everything*. I'm not going to dwell on those traits here because they really don't discriminate between people who have different kinds of fantasies—these are traits that, for the most part, simply predispose us to having more fantasies in general about a wide range of content. These include having an overactive imagination, possessing a strong sex drive, having very favorable attitudes toward sex, having a preference for thrilling and risky sexual experiences, having an easy time separating sex from emotion, and being open to trying new things in general. All of these traits are linked to more fantasies about the seven major themes we identified earlier in this book, with few exceptions.

One final point before we get to our fifteen-question countdown: when it comes to the factors that predict our sex fantasies, we don't always know for sure which came first, the trait or the fantasy. Because we're dealing with correlational data here, we cannot make definitive cause-and-effect statements. As a result, while I've framed this chapter from the perspective of how your personal traits may predispose you to having certain fantasies, I'm mindful of the limitations of the data, which is why you'll see me make frequent mention of this chicken-and-egg problem.

1. How Old Are You?

Age is one of the most common and superficial things we ask each other about in casual conversation—but it turns out that the answer may reveal something much deeper. In fact, our age says a lot about our sexual desires, but not necessarily in the way you might expect. For example, you might be tempted to think that the younger someone is, the more interested that person would be in threesomes. I mean, if anyone wants a three-way, it's college-age adults, right? Not so fast. The results of my survey suggest that the college crowd is the *least* likely to be interested in threesomes, and there's actually a very good reason for this.

As you'll see throughout this chapter, our sexual fantasies appear to be carefully designed to meet our psychological needs—and because those needs change and evolve over our life span, it seems that our sexual fantasies naturally adjust in order to accommodate them. Rather than being static, our sexual fantasies should therefore be thought of as undergoing a developmental process that unfolds as we enter new stages of life.

To better understand this idea, let's do a little perspective-taking exercise. I'm going to generalize a bit here, but please bear with me. First, put yourself in the shoes of a horny college student for a moment. At this age, sex itself is still a novelty because you haven't been doing it very long (after all, the average age of first intercourse is sixteen to seventeen). You also haven't yet had a very wide range of sexual partners or experiences. At the same time, you're at the peak of sexual insecurity—you're worried about what other people think regarding both your appearance and sexual performance. And on top of all that, you're embedded in a hookup culture that pushes short-term sexual flings over dating.

Now, let's swap shoes with someone at middle age. You sowed your wild oats in your twenties, experiencing several partners, activities, and sensations along the way. Sex is no longer new—you've been doing it for decades, perhaps over and over again with the same partner because you've settled down. You've also reached the glorious "zero fucks" stage of life, meaning you've realized that life is too short to spend it in a perpetual state of anxiety about what other people think.

There's a world of difference when it comes to what turns someone on at these life stages. My survey results revealed that, compared to older adults, younger adults were less likely to fantasize about group sex, nonmonogamy, novelty, and taboo acts. This pattern makes perfect sense because for young adults, sex—*any* opportunity for sex—is novel and exciting, even if it's just with one partner and doesn't involve any, ahem, adventuresome activities. In other words, young adults largely appear to be content with basic sex, no need for bells and whistles. By contrast, older adults—especially those in long-term, monogamous relationships—are more likely to crave something fresh and new, something that's going to put the Coolidge Effect in check, like an orgy or an open relationship.

At the same time, younger adults were more likely to report fantasies about BDSM and passion/romance than those who were older. This also makes sense, but for a different reason—it's due to that difference in insecurity. Younger people were more likely to say their sexual fantasies were designed to help them escape reality, to reduce anxiety, and to help them feel more sexually confident. Fantasies of BDSM and passion can be helpful in accomplishing these goals. For example, fantasizing about being dominant or in control could help to bolster one's feelings of confidence, whereas fantasies about passion could blunt feelings of sexual insecurity or inadequacy.

One other interesting way that sexual fantasies are related to age is that sexual flexibility fantasies are more common among older than younger men. Most notably, the older heterosexual guys in my sample were increasingly likely to report same-sex fantasies. By contrast, women's sexual flexibility fantasies were unrelated to their age. This pattern fits in well with the idea that women have more sexual flexibility than men to begin with—but it also suggests the provocative possibility that some men might grow into their flexibility with age. Or maybe it's just a sign that, as men age and have more opportunities to fantasize, the content of their fantasies simply becomes more and more diverse.

2. What Is Your Sexual Orientation?

For years, psychologists have told us that, aside from the gender of the people in our fantasies, our sexual orientation has little—and perhaps nothing—to do with the content of our fantasies. My survey results suggest that this conclusion is wrong—very, very wrong. Our sexual orientation actually speaks volumes about our desires.

Broadly speaking, what I found was that people who identified as anything other than heterosexual were more likely to fantasize about sexual freedom in numerous forms. Specifically, nonheterosexuals were more likely to fantasize about BDSM, nonmonogamy, taboo acts, and gender-bending. If you think about it, the common denominator for all of these interests is that they involve breaking free of cultural rules or constraints for how we should act or behave. Therefore, one potential explanation is simply that having a nonheterosexual orientation predisposes one to developing these other interests because breaking one sexual taboo makes it less costly to violate others. Think about it this way: if you already know that other people aren't going to accept your relationship because of your partner's gender, shucking monogamy or other sexual conventions doesn't really incur any extra costs. However, we have the classic chicken-and-egg problem here—we don't know which sexual interest came first. In other words, does having same-sex attraction increase the odds of having taboo fantasies? Or does having taboo fantasies in general increase the likelihood of acknowledging same-sex attractions, leading to the adoption of alternative sexual identity labels? I'd wager that both explanations are true to an extent.

I should also clarify that the link between nonheterosexuality and taboo desires reflects, to some degree, the fact that persons who are strongly attracted to a specific taboo often find that traditional sexual orientation labels don't accurately capture their interests. Therefore, they sometimes choose alternative labels that have nothing to do with the gender of their partners but rather reflect the nature of their taboo interests, such as the handful of survey participants who, when asked for their sexual orientation, wrote in "pedophile" or "zoophile," labels that denote attraction to children and animals, respectively.

3. Do You Have a Religious Affiliation?

Most major religions places constraints on their followers' sexual behaviors, specifying not just who they're allowed to have sex with—usually, a spouse and no one else—but also what they're allowed to do—namely, utilitarian penile-vaginal intercourse with the goal of making babies. Interestingly, what I found in my survey was that people who were religiously affiliated and who, presumably, had the most sexual constraints placed upon them, tended to fantasize more about breaking free of them. Specifically, they were more likely to fantasize about a range of novel and taboo sex acts. They seemed to be demonstrating what psychologists call *reactance*, the idea that when our perceived freedoms are threatened or when we're pressured to adopt a certain view or attitude, we respond in a way that's opposite of what the authority or requestor wants.[1] In other words, rather than getting in line, we rebel. Incidentally, this is why so-called reverse psychology works so well— instead of working against reactance, you can use it in your favor by asking someone to do the opposite of what you really want them to do.

In contrast to novelty and taboo fantasies, reactance was not evident in gender-bending: religiously affiliated persons were actually *less* likely to fantasize about breaking free of culturally imposed gender roles. This suggests that religiously affiliated folks tend to buy into traditional ideas of what men and women are supposed to be and that this carries over into the content of their sexual fantasies. Interestingly, though, while the religiously affiliated were less likely to fantasize about gender-bending, they were more likely to fantasize about sexual flexibility—at least the men were. Specifically, heterosexual guys who were religiously affiliated were more likely to have gay fantasies than men who lacked a religious affiliation. To me, this suggests that reactance isn't the whole story here. Perhaps people who have fantasies they want to change or fantasies they feel are wrong sometimes seek out religion in order to cope. So maybe the link between heterosexual men's same-sex fantasies and having a religious affiliation is more a function of some of these guys hoping to "pray the gay away." (Which, as it turns out, doesn't really work, according to science.[2])

One other type of fantasy linked to religiosity involved meeting emotional needs: religiously affiliated persons were more likely to fantasize about intimacy and social bonding. This

suggests that religious people tend to see sex and emotional fulfillment as intertwined—a concept embedded in many religious
teachings—with two people coming together body and soul. In
sum, the fantasies of religious folks adhere to traditional notions of gender and the idea that sex and love go together, but
they also stand in defiance to mandates that sex should only
comprise a narrow range of acts.

4. Are You a Democrat or Republican?

Our political affiliations tell a story that's fairly similar to the
one told by our religious affiliations.

Despite being the party that claims to offer the staunchest
support of individual liberty and freedom, the Republican Party
espouses a pretty limited view of what is acceptable when it
comes to sex: sex should be reserved for the context of a lifelong monogamous marriage, because its primary purpose is
making a family. Activities that prioritize pleasure over pro-
creation, like nonmonogamy and kinky sexual practices, are
frowned upon. Nowhere are these views more evident than in
Republican politicians' insistence on pushing for abstinence-
until-marriage sex education. Perhaps not surprisingly, research
has found that Republicans tend to have a more limited sexual
repertoire than do Democrats. Specifically, Republicans are
more likely to report engaging in traditional sexual behaviors
like missionary-style penile-vaginal intercourse, whereas Democrats are more likely to say they have experimented with riskier
and more adventuresome sexual activities.[3]

Interestingly, however, what the Republican Party stands for
when it comes to sex and what Republicans say they're doing

in the bedroom isn't reflected in their fantasies. I found that Republicans fantasized more about most of the things they aren't supposed to want than did Democrats. Specifically, Republicans were more likely to fantasize about both nonmonogamous sex—in particular, orgies, infidelity, swinging, and cuckolding— as well as taboo activities like exhibitionism, voyeurism, and fetishism. Like religion, politics seems to be another case where there's a bit of reactance taking place: we come to want what the political authorities tell us we can't have.

That said, there were a few things Democrats fantasized about more than Republicans. For instance, Democrats were more likely to fantasize about BDSM, as well as intimacy and social bonding. This pattern of results suggests that sexual fantasies could potentially take on a different meaning for people depending on their political affiliations: whereas Republicans' fantasies are more likely to focus on novel sex acts seemingly because they have more restrictions placed on what they can do in real life, Democrats—who don't face the same restrictions—are more likely to fantasize about meeting specific psychological needs, such as escaping self-awareness (in the case of BDSM fantasies) or feeling validated and loved (in the case of intimacy fantasies).

One other fantasy related to party affiliation was genderbending: Democrats were more likely to have gender-bending fantasies than Republicans. This is another chicken-and-egg case: Do people with gender-bending interests gravitate toward political parties that are likely to be more accepting of them, or does being part of a political party that espouses ideals of gender equality allow people the freedom to acknowledge gendervariant interests? This is another case where I suspect there's a bit of both going on.

5. What Was Your First Sexual Experience Like?

Some research suggests that our first sexual experience is the most important in the sense that it sets the tone for our future sex lives. For example, people who look back on the loss of their virginity favorably tend to find their current sex lives to be more satisfying.[4] Findings like this made me wonder whether and how the specific activities that took place during one's first sexual experience are related to the kinds of things that one currently fantasizes about. My survey results revealed that if a specific sex act took place during one's very first sexual experience—be it kissing, oral sex, penile-vaginal intercourse, or something else—people fantasized about it more frequently as adults. In addition, people who said that their first sexual experience was unusual in some way tended to report more unusual sexual fantasies throughout their lives, meaning their fantasies were less likely to follow the cultural script for how sex is "supposed" to happen. Specifically, I found that an unusual first experience was linked to more fantasies about BDSM, taboo sex acts, gender-bending, and emotionless sex. Why is that? Well, if your first experience is unusual—but still a positive experience overall—that might give you a broader outlook on what's acceptable when it comes to sex while simultaneously reinforcing the idea that kinky sex is pleasurable. When we're young and inexperienced, we don't have as much of an idea about what "normal" sexual behavior is, so our lived experiences have the potential to profoundly shape our sense of normalcy going forward.

It's also interesting to note that, among my participants who said a taboo act was their favorite fantasy of all time, one in eight said this fantasy stemmed from an actual childhood sexual experience. This provides an interesting contrast to participants whose favorite fantasies were, say, group sex and novelty because these folks were far more likely to say that their fantasies stemmed from sexual experiences they had as adults. All of this is simply to say that when we have an unusual first sexual experience, it has the potential to imprint on us in a way that we carry forward for the rest of our lives. Again, though, it's also possible that our current desires influence what we remember from our sexual histories and/or the significance we attach to those early experiences.

6. Have You Ever Been the Victim of a Sex Crime?

Of course, your first sexual experience isn't the only one that matters in understanding what you fantasize about and why. My survey results suggest that people's experiences with sexual victimization matter a lot, too—a conclusion that I suspect will prove quite controversial. I asked my participants if they had ever been the victim of any kind of sex crime, and it turned out that approximately one in ten men and two in five women had. These disturbing figures may strike some readers as unusually high, generating concern that victims are disproportionately overrepresented in my data. However, the question I asked was very broad, meaning "sex crime" could indicate any number of things, including but not limited to harassment, sexual assault, and indecent exposure. When you consider that national US surveys and polls have found that as many as one in ten men and one in four women have been sexually harassed in the workplace and that harassment is just one of many possible sex crimes, it appears that the rate at which my participants reported experiencing sex crimes is, sadly, quite typical.[5]

Those who had been sexually victimized fantasized more often about a whole host of things, but before we get into them, let me be abundantly clear: the fantasies we're going to talk about here are not inherently pathological, nor are they necessarily signs that someone has psychological problems. To the contrary, as you'll see below, I argue that these fantasies are adaptive coping mechanisms for dealing with previous sexual trauma and, if anything, should be viewed as a sign of psychological resilience.

With that said, victims of sex crimes were more likely than nonvictims to fantasize about almost all aspects of BDSM (dominance being the primary exception), both emotional (passion, romance, and intimacy) *and* emotionless sex, gender-bending, and sexual flexibility. Let's explore each of these in turn.

First, the BDSM finding was truly surprising to me because other published studies have found no link between previous experiences with sexual victimization and BDSM.[6] However, I think this discrepancy is attributable to the fact that most prior studies examined how victimization is related to the actual *practice* of BDSM, not BDSM fantasies. In other words, victimization may play a role in whether people are likely to fantasize about BDSM but not necessarily in whether they try it in real life. That said, the associations here were small, and most people who reported BDSM fantasies had *not* been victims of sex crimes—so whatever role victimization might play here is a very small one. However, it makes sense from the standpoint that BDSM offers distraction and an escape from self-awareness—a way of losing oneself in the moment. It's important to note that those who identified as victims reported lower self-esteem, more anxiety, and more sexual problems, which tells us that we're talking about a group of people who may be especially in need of distraction—they need to redirect attention away from negative thoughts and feelings that might diminish their arousal. To be clear, this is not about people wanting to relive past abuse; rather, it's far more plausible that this is a psychological coping mechanism through which *some* people may learn to temporarily alleviate anxiety stemming from prior victimization.

Second, the fact that victims were more likely to fantasize about both emotional and emotionless sex might seem paradoxical at first; however, I believe it reflects the fact that different people cope with sexual victimization in different ways. As mentioned above, victims of sex crimes often experience a lingering psychological impact that is very negative, including low self-esteem, anxiety, and depression. In order to cope with this, some victims may fantasize about sexual encounters that affirm and validate their self-worth. By contrast, however, other victims may try to buffer their feelings of self-worth by checking their emotions at the door entirely and focusing only on the sex act itself in their fantasies.

Finally, the links between sexual victimization and fantasies about gender-bending and sexual flexibility could be explained in at least two ways. One possibility is simply that people who are more willing to disclose stigmatized sexual interests are more likely to disclose other potentially stigmatizing aspects of their sex lives, including experiences with sexual violence. This explanation suggests that there's no deeper meaning to these associations and that self-disclosure is the common denominator.

However, we might also be talking about coping mechanisms here. For example, research has found that experiences with rape and sexual abuse sometimes lead to self-hatred and/or disgust with one's own body, and this, in turn, may stimulate attempts to psychologically escape or dissociate from one's own body. One example would be fantasizing about becoming the other sex.[7] To be clear, this is not to suggest that transsexualism is inherently rooted in sexual abuse. Let me be emphatic about this: *it's not*. Rather, the point is simply that gender-bending fantasies are one potential means by which a small number of people might learn to cope with a reality of past abuse.

As for sexual-flexibility fantasies, I found that women who identified as exclusively lesbian were more likely to report fantasies involving men to the extent that they had been sexually victimized. To me, this suggests the possibility that sexual victimization could potentially influence the sexual identity labels that women with same-sex attractions adopt. For instance, a bisexual woman who is victimized by a man might subsequently adopt a lesbian identity, perhaps because disidentifying with her attraction to men provides a psychological sense of safety or relief. Thus, both sexual identity and sexual fantasy content have the potential to serve as coping mechanisms for sexual abuse in some cases.

Let me reiterate that the links between sexual victimization and sexual fantasies were small, owing to the fact that victimization can take many different forms and not everyone copes in the same way. Also, let me repeat that these associations should not be taken to mean that any of these fantasies are inherently pathological or that everyone who has them has been sexually abused. The key takeaway here is that some of the most common sexual fantasies have the potential to help people cope with previous sexual traumas, which speaks to the powerful role that our fantasies can play in shaping our sexual well-being.

7. Are You Currently Experiencing Any Sexual Problems?

Beyond serving as potential coping mechanisms for survivors of sexual abuse, sexual fantasies can be seen as coping mechanisms for sexual difficulties more broadly. For example, my survey results revealed that people who had problems with sexual desire, arousal, and orgasm were more likely to fantasize about BDSM acts. Just as we discussed above in the context of previous victimization, BDSM may be appealing fantasy content to anyone looking to block out feelings of anxiety and insecurity that might otherwise interfere with their ability to relax and enjoy sex. Likewise, having sexual problems was linked to more fantasies about emotional sex—specifically, seeking intimacy and approval. These feelings of validation might be useful not just for bolstering self-esteem but also for putting one's mind at ease more generally.

Interestingly, persons with more sex problems reported fewer fantasies about novelty, group sex, and nonmonogamy. However, this makes sense when you consider that the goal for persons with sexual difficulties is usually just having sex—novelty isn't necessarily what they need and might even be counterproductive. After all, novelty introduces an element of the unexpected and can potentially be stressful, which might exacerbate any problems one might be experiencing.

Lastly, I also found that persons with sexual problems were more likely to fantasize about taboo acts. On the one hand, like BDSM, this might reflect a search for distraction and escape. On the other hand, however, it might also reflect the fact that people with sexual difficulties tend to be drawn to the taboo because when people have problems establishing the kinds of sexual relationships they want, they're more likely to gravitate toward unusual sexual activities in order to seek fulfillment.

8. Do You Have Compulsive Sexual Urges?

There's a big difference between having a high sex drive and having compulsive sexual urges. A high sex drive simply means that you find yourself wanting sex frequently; however, it's all under your control and it's not affecting you or your relationship(s) negatively. By contrast, compulsive sexual urges are desires that you find yourself struggling to control—they are distressing urges that get in the way of your everyday life and/or your ability to establish the kind of relationship(s) you want.

My survey results revealed that people with high sex drives fantasized more about almost everything. Interestingly, though, that wasn't the case for those with compulsive urges. People who said they have compulsive desires were really only more likely to fantasize about emotionless sex, taboo sex acts, and gender-bending. As we discussed earlier, labeling one's desires as "compulsive" or "out of control" often signifies underlying moral conflicts. (Incidentally, saying one's sexual desires are "out of control" is also a strategy frequently used by rich and powerful men who want to absolve themselves of personal responsibility when they're caught behaving badly—but that's a whole other story.) So part of what we're seeing here may just be that a lot of people who fantasize about emotionless sex, taboo activities, and gender-bending simply feel guilty about desiring these things. Consistent with this idea, I found that fantasies about these three acts were linked to reporting more feelings of sexual shame. That said, I want to be clear that compulsive desires aren't always about moral conflicts or deflecting blame. Some folks legitimately have issues regulating and controlling their sexual urges irrespective of the perceived morality of their sexual desires, and they may benefit from professional help in managing them.

I should also mention that the link between compulsive sexual tendencies and fantasies about taboo acts in particular might partially reflect the fact that persons with obsessive-compulsive disorder (OCD) sometimes present with obsessions and compulsions about unusual sex acts.[8] Specifically, what we're talking about here are cases in which a taboo desire takes on a ritualistic nature in which there's a certain trigger of fear or anxiety that can only be relieved by a very specific (and often taboo) sexual practice. For example, a compulsive male exhibitionist might engage in ritualized flashing of unsuspecting female strangers as a way of coping with his feelings of sexual inadequacy. Every time he experiences these feelings, he may feel compelled to start flashing because it's the only way he has learned to relieve those feelings. To be clear, not all taboo sexual interests are variants of OCD; however, they sometimes are, and it's important to recognize this because it has significant implications for treatment.

Interestingly, some studies have also found a link between OCD and gender dysphoria—that is, the feeling that one is trapped in the body of the wrong sex.[9] In these cases, people may have intrusive thoughts that they are transgender, despite the fact that they aren't actually transgender. This creates anxiety that one may try to resolve by engaging in any number of compulsive activities, such as repeatedly checking one's genitals or frequently seeking reassurance from others about one's gender identity. To be perfectly clear, this is not to suggest that transgenderism and OCD are one and the same—they aren't, not by a long shot. It's important to clearly distinguish them in the interest of ensuring appropriate treatment and assistance, such as determining who is and is not a candidate for gender-affirmation surgery. I simply mention the OCD–gender dysphoria association because it may be a small part of the reason why gender-bending fantasies were specifically linked to compulsive sexual urges among my participants, whereas most other fantasies were not.

9. How Do You Feel About Your Current Relationship?

The way people feel about their current relationship—including how happy they are and how much power they hold relative to their partner—seems to be reflected in many different kinds of sexual fantasies. First, I found that the less happy people were with their relationships, the more likely they were to fantasize about having an open or polyamorous relationship and committing infidelity, as well as both emotional (passion, romance, and intimacy) and emotionless sex.

Of course, it shouldn't be surprising that unhappy people were more likely to fantasize about having sex with someone other than their current partner—but in these fantasies, they seemed content to do it regardless of whether they had their partner's consent or not. Interestingly, however, being unhappy with one's relationship was unrelated to swinging and cuckolding fantasies, which tells us that low satisfaction doesn't necessarily mean someone is interested in nonmonogamy across the board—instead, they're primarily interested in the forms of nonmonogamy that don't involve their partner's direct sexual participation. They really just want to be with someone else for a change.

The emotional and emotionless sex findings might seem paradoxical at first, but—as we discussed above in the section on sexual victimization—these dual associations might reflect differences in coping strategies. For example, some people might be fantasizing about passion and romance because it reflects the kind of relationship they yearn to have with their partner. Perhaps this even provides some feeling of reassurance that things might eventually change. It's also possible that these emotional fantasies are signs that people are mentally working through their relationship problems and searching for solutions. By contrast, others might keep their emotions at bay in their fantasies as a form of self-protection. Think about it this way: if there's no emotion present, then their already-hurt feelings cannot be hurt any further.

In sum, when people aren't happy with their relationship, they may use their fantasies as a way of escaping problems, correcting problems, or protecting their own feelings. Of course, there's also a bit of the chicken-and-egg issue here: Does being in an unhappy relationship lead people to have these fantasies, or does having these fantasies potentially harm people's relationships? We can't rule out the possibility that there's a bit of both going on here. For instance, if someone already has doubts about whether their partner is right for them, it's possible that certain kinds of fantasies—like infidelity—could exacerbate those doubts.

Relationship power was also related to fantasy content, but really only to BDSM fantasies. However, the association I found probably isn't the one that you might expect. Specifically, those who reported having more power tended to have more fantasies about dominance and sadism, whereas those with less power fantasized more about submission and masochism. Thus, although you may have previously heard that people with power use their fantasies to escape its burden, that doesn't seem to be the case. While that may be true for a small number of individuals, generally speaking, people's sexual fantasies tend to reflect the amount of power they currently have in their relationship.

10. What Is Your Attachment Style?

The degree to which you feel insecure in your relationship says a lot about the kinds of things you are—and aren't—likely to fantasize about. By "insecure," I mean feeling like you need a lot of reassurance that your partner loves you and worrying that your partner might abandon you. I found that the more insecure people said they were, the less likely they were to fantasize about group sex and nonmonogamy and the more likely they were to fantasize about BDSM, sexual novelty, and romance.

The fact that insecure people had fewer fantasies about multiple partners and nonmonogamy is perfectly logical. Insecure people are likely to find these scenarios threatening because there's the potential for jealousy to set in if, say, you see your partner giving attention to someone other than you, or if someone else appears to be taken with your partner. To the extent that insecure people do fantasize about group sex or nonmonogamy (and some of them certainly do), they tend to place themselves at the center of attention, perhaps so as to minimize feelings of threat. An insecure person might very much enjoy a scenario in which multiple people are vying for their attention because that blunts any potential feelings of rejection. As this example illustrates, with a little creative thinking, people can tailor virtually any fantasy scenario to meet their needs.

The link between insecurity and fantasies about BDSM and novelty can be explained as a form of psychological escapism. As previously mentioned, BDSM fantasies in particular offer a break from self-awareness—but novelty fantasies do as well. I found that having frequent novelty fantasies was linked to saying that one uses fantasies in general as a means of reducing anxiety and escaping reality during sex. In other words, both BDSM and novelty are potent ways of taking your mind off of relationship insecurities.

Finally, the link between insecurity and romance may stem from the fact that people who are insecure find it difficult to enjoy sex—including the very thought of it—unless they feel desired and validated. Therefore, anxious folks might actively include calming emotional content in their fantasies as a way of helping them to relax and get in the mood. Consistent with this idea, the participants who reported having more of these emotion-based fantasies were also the most likely to say that the reason they fantasize in the first place is to relieve anxiety.

11. Are You Someone Who Is Organized and Cares About the Details?

People who are high in the personality trait of conscientiousness tend to be pretty detail-oriented and organized in their everyday life—and this appears to transfer over into their sexual fantasies. Being conscientious was linked to having more novelty fantasies, especially fantasies that featured novel settings. It appears that their attention to detail may lead conscientious persons to construct elaborate fantasies that are planned down to the location where the activity takes place.

At the same time, conscientious folks were less likely to fantasize about BDSM, taboo acts, and gender-bending. This pattern makes sense when you consider that conscientious persons like to follow the rules—they tend to be conformists. As such, they're probably less aroused by the idea of engaging in activities that are seen as culturally forbidden or, in the case of gender-bending, that might make the world seem like a less orderly and predictable place.

12. Would You Describe Yourself as Outgoing and Sociable?

Extraversion is a personality trait that reflects an outgoing nature, a desire to interact with the world. Extraverts like to meet new people in real life—and in their sexual fantasies, too. I found that extraversion was linked to more fantasies about group sex, as well as more fantasies about both consensual nonmonogamy and infidelity. This isn't at all surprising, because being socially confident probably makes it a lot easier to imagine meeting and seducing new partners. Extraverts also tend to have more novelty fantasies, which can be seen as another symptom of their greater tendency to engage with the world around them.

By the same token, extraverts were less likely to have taboo sexual fantasies. This fits with the finding that people who have difficulty establishing the kinds of relationships they want tend to generate more unusual interests. Extraverts usually don't have a problem establishing relationships, so it makes sense that the taboo would hold less appeal to them.

Extraversion was also linked to the emotional content in one's fantasies. Specifically, extraverts had fewer fantasies about intimacy and social bonding and more fantasies about feeling validated. In particular, extraverts had more fantasies about being praised for their sexual skills and performance, meaning their fantasies were more likely to center around boosting their egos than they were around developing deep emotional connections with others. I guess the way to think about this is that extraverts don't just want to be seen as the life of the party—they also want to be seen as the life of the *sex* party.

13. How Much Do You Care About Other People's Problems?

The personality trait of agreeableness is characterized by a high degree of care and concern for others. Agreeable people are kind, considerate, and willing to sacrifice their own self-interest when necessary. Perhaps not surprisingly, their sexual fantasies reflect their inherently prosocial nature. For example, I found that the more agreeable people were, the less likely they were to have fantasies about infidelity, BDSM, emotionless sex, and taboo sex acts, especially taboo acts that were nonconsensual (like sex with children and animals). In other words, agreeable people don't seem to find it arousing to fantasize about sex acts in which someone would get hurt or—in the case of BDSM—where there might be pain involved, even if that pain is desired. In the case of emotionless sex, agreeable people probably aren't into it because in the absence of intimacy, it might not be clear to them whether the other person is enjoying sex.

By contrast, agreeable persons were more likely to fantasize about novel sex acts, as well as one specific form of consensual nonmonogamy: swinging. I interpret this as meaning that agreeable persons tend to fantasize about things they think will make others happy, such as trying a new sex toy that their partner might like or, with respect to swinging, watching one's partner have their sexual needs fulfilled by someone else. In other words, agreeable persons tend to fantasize only about new activities that they think will be mutually enjoyable.

14. How Well Do You Handle Stress?

Neuroticism is a personality trait characterized by emotional instability. Neurotics don't cope with stress very well and tend to have very negative reactions toward it. In light of this, it shouldn't be surprising that neurotic people tend to play it safe when it comes to their sexual fantasies, reporting fewer fantasies about group sex, nonmonogamy, and novelty. They don't express much desire for new activities or new partners because they don't necessarily know what they're getting. That uncertainty can be stressful, especially when coupled with the prospect of a partner potentially expressing interest in someone else, such as in the case of a threesome. Instead, they seem to prefer more predictable sexual interactions that follow an established script.

What neurotics do tend to fantasize about are BDSM and passion/romance. This tells us that their fantasies tend to be about either distraction and escape or calming emotional content. Either way, the goal seems to be fending off feelings of stress and insecurity.

15. How Do You Feel About Yourself?

Lastly, I found that self-esteem, the degree to which one holds a positive or negative self-view, was related to fantasy content in numerous ways. Specifically, the lower someone's self-esteem, the more likely they were to fantasize about passion/romance and taboo sex acts. This pattern suggests that, just like neurotic and insecure people, those with low self-esteem often fantasize about receiving reassurance and validation. This can be seen as a self-protective strategy of sorts that buffers one's self-image against further hits. It also suggests that, like introverts and people suffering from sexual problems, those who are lacking in self-confidence may gravitate to more unusual sexual desires due to difficulties starting the kinds of sexual relationships they want.

Low self-esteem was also linked to more fantasies about BDSM, a finding that was initially surprising to me in light of previous research suggesting that people who practice BDSM are just as psychologically healthy as the rest of the population, if not more so.[10] However, I think there's a logical explanation for these seemingly discrepant findings. Before I get into that, though, let's be clear about one thing: it is emphatically *not* the case that everyone who is into BDSM is "fifty shades of fucked up," as author E. L. James's books might lead you to believe. The association here, though statistically significant, was small, which tells us that most of the people who have BDSM fantasies are perfectly well-adjusted. So why were my findings a little different? The studies linking BDSM to positive psychological adjustment recruited participants from BDSM clubs or interest groups. These were individuals who were therefore already acting on their fantasies, had a social network of like-minded people, and had made BDSM a part of their personal identity. By contrast, I didn't specifically recruit people who were living in the BDSM scene. Instead, I looked at *anyone* who reported having BDSM fantasies, regardless of whether they had acted on them—and most of my participants had not done so.

Interestingly, I found that my participants who *had* acted on their BDSM fantasies reported higher self-esteem, fewer feelings of guilt and shame, and better psychological adjustment than those who hadn't. What this tells us is that the discrepancy between my findings and the other studies out there would appear to be, at least in part, a function of the fact that I'm studying the fantasy whereas others are studying the reality. I think there's an interesting parallel one could draw here to homosexuality and mental health: gay and lesbian persons who aren't out about their sexual orientation often have a high degree of internalized homophobia or self-hatred. The more of this self-hatred one has, the more one's mental health tends to suffer.[11] By contrast, those who learn to love themselves, who become actively involved in the gay community, and who find social acceptance—they thrive. Therefore, feeling ashamed of a sexual desire—whether it involves same-sex attraction, BDSM, or something else—can be harmful, whereas coming to terms with and accepting one's desires can enhance well-being. Remember this point because we'll return to it a little later in the book when we consider the steps necessary for acceptance of one's fantasies.

One final linkage I found between self-esteem and fantasy content was that persons with higher self-esteem were more likely to fantasize about consensual nonmonogamy. Thus, people who feel positive about themselves are more likely to imagine being in sexually open relationships, whereas those who hold negative self-views are more likely to fantasize about monogamy. This—combined with the insecurity findings mentioned above—suggests that you need a certain amount of self-confidence to feel comfortable envisioning yourself in an open relationship. Those with a poor self-image may find the prospect of nonmonogamy to be either too unrealistic (because they simply can't envision more than one person being attracted to them) or threatening (because they fear their partner might decide to leave them for someone else). Of course, it's probably also true that having multiple partners who desire you enhances self-esteem.

So What Do These Fifteen Questions Tell Us?

In this chapter, we explored fifteen questions whose answers say something about our sexual desires. The survey findings that we discussed suggest that our demographic backgrounds, sexual histories, and personality traits all come together to create a unique set of psychological needs—needs that are reflected in our sexual fantasies. Remember that these needs and the fantasies that mirror them are not necessarily static over the course of our lives. Life circumstances, such as new relationships and new sexual experiences, can reshape our needs time and again, which means that our fantasies have the potential to "reset" periodically. As a result, you're in good company if you've found that the things you fantasize about now aren't the same things you were fantasizing about, say, in high school.

Let me reiterate that it's shortsighted to try to understand someone's sexual fantasies by looking at single traits in isolation; instead, we must consider a combination of multiple traits and what the overall pattern reveals. For example, if you only knew someone's age, you probably wouldn't have a very accurate picture of what that person's fantasies are likely to be. However, if you also knew this person's level of self-esteem, attachment style, and personality profile, you could probably generate a much clearer picture, especially if several of those traits point in the direction of the same fantasy. For instance, being younger, having low self-esteem, and being high in neuroticism and insecurity are all linked to more fantasies about BDSM and fewer fantasies about nonmonogamy.

I should also repeat that, while our psychological needs shape our fantasies, our fantasies also have the potential to shape how we view ourselves, how we interpret our sexual histories, and how we feel about our relationships. In other words, it goes both ways.

Up until this point, we've primarily focused on *what* we fantasize about doing—and what this says about us. But what about the specific partners we envision having in our fantasies? Who are they? And what the heck does that say about us? These are the questions we'll explore next.

5

Tell Me Who *You Want*

Who Are We Fantasizing About? How Do We See Ourselves in Our Fantasies? And What Does It All Mean?

Rather than focusing on *what* we're doing in our sexual fantasies, this chapter will focus on *who* we're doing, as well as how we see ourselves. We'll first consider how Americans describe their ideal sex partner. What kinds of body and genital characteristics does this person have? And how are these preferences shaped by our gender, sexual orientation, race, personality, and porn-use habits? As you'll soon see, the bodies we tend to picture in our fantasies say a lot about us—and our culture.

Next, we'll talk about the specific people who appear in our fantasies. How often do we fantasize about our romantic partners as opposed to celebrities, porn stars, politicians, and superheroes? Which famous faces are most likely to appear in our fantasies? And does it matter who we're fantasizing about, anyway? Yes—it turns out that the people who populate our fantasies say something important about the way our current sex lives and relationships are going.

Last, we'll explore the ways in which we change ourselves in our fantasies. How many of us alter our body, personality, or age? Do men and women change themselves in similar or different ways when they fantasize? And what does it say about us if there's a big discrepancy between our fantasy selves and our actual selves? Quite a lot, as you'll see.

What Women (and Men) Want

In order to fully appreciate the significance of what our fantasy partners look like, we first need to establish a reference point. So let's take a peek at what the body of the typical American looks like. The average adult man is five feet nine inches tall and weighs 196 pounds.[1] His body mass index (BMI)—a ratio of height to weight that's commonly used to determine whether someone is under- or overweight—is 28.7, a figure that puts him squarely in the "overweight" category (a "normal" BMI is generally considered to be between 18.5 and 25). Likewise, the average adult woman is five feet four inches tall and weighs 169 pounds.[2] Her BMI is 29.2, which means that she's also overweight according to medical standards.

So how do our fantasy partners' body proportions compare to those of the average American?

The Dreamboat: Straight Women's Fantasy Man
The straight women who took my survey described the men in their fantasies as tall and hunky: on average, they were six feet tall and weighed 182 pounds. This translates to a BMI of 24.7, a number that would fall into the "normal" category. In other words, the guys walking around in women's heads are far taller

and fitter than they are in reality. Indeed, a guy who is six feet tall would be in the 85th percentile for height, which further highlights just how far from average these fantasy dudes are! To be clear, however, while women are largely fantasizing about tall men with athletic bodies, they don't necessarily want guys who are overly built—less than one in ten women described the men in their fantasies as "very muscular," meaning they're not usually picturing the muscle-bound hunks we see so often on cinema screens.

Women describe their typical fantasy partners as, in addition to being fit, having brown or black hair. They also say he's done a bit of manscaping but hasn't removed all of his body hair. Just 4 percent said they prefer a man who shaves his entire body, while 3 percent said they prefer a guy who does no trimming at all. As far as his pubic hair grooming is concerned, the numbers were similar, with most imagining a guy who keeps things under control but hasn't removed everything.

Women also fantasize about men who are more well-endowed than average. The guys in women's fantasies have an average erect penis length of 6.9 inches. By contrast, studies suggest that the average erect penis length in the real world is just over 5 inches.[3] However, asking women to report inches desired in the abstract is likely to generate overestimates. I say this because in a study where women were given a series of life-size penis models and asked to pick out their ideal, the average model selected was closer to 6 inches.[4] Either way, however, these numbers suggest that straight women think the optimal penis is a little larger than average. Most women also said that they primarily fantasize about circumcised men (just one in ten fantasize only about uncircumcised guys). This isn't surprising in light of the fact that most men in the United States have had their foreskin removed, so that's probably what American women are used to seeing.

To sum it up, straight women in America tend to fantasize about tall, dark, and handsome guys with larger-than-average penises who are "metrosexuals" in the sense that they do some regular body and pubic hair grooming.

The Perfect 10: Straight Men's Fantasy Woman

So how do heterosexual men picture their fantasy woman? In terms of height, they fantasize about women who are five feet five inches tall, which is only one inch taller than the average American woman. This tells us not only that guys' height preferences are grounded in reality but also that men tend to be drawn to women who are shorter than they are. Weight is another story, though. The women in men's fantasies weigh just 131 pounds on average—that's only about 75 percent of what women in the real world weigh. These fantasy women have a BMI of 21.8, which is at the low end of normal; however, it's not exactly in the supermodel-thin category. For comparison purposes, the average female supermodel weighs just 118 pounds, but she's also six inches taller than the average American woman, giving her a very underweight BMI of 16.9.[5] So when you factor in both desired height *and* desired weight, the women in men's fantasies are somewhere in between supermodel and average—they're very close to average in terms of height and closer to supermodel than average in terms of weight.

While we've all heard that "gentlemen prefer blondes," just one-quarter of men said their fantasy woman has golden hair. Twice as many said that she's a brunette. In addition, these fantasy women don't have any body hair and their pubic hair is either completely gone or there's only a very small amount present, such as a so-called landing strip. Just 3 percent of the straight men who took my survey expressed a desire for a full bush, meaning no pubic hair removal at all.

Admittedly, there isn't a great way to capture the size of the breasts that men fantasize about because guys don't tend to think about their desired bust size in terms of inches and they don't have much experience guesstimating this. So what I ended up doing instead was asking them to choose the bra cup size that most closely matches the size of the breasts they fantasize about on a scale ranging from AA (labeled as "very small") to DDD+ (labeled as "very large"), with C being right in the middle. On average, guys said that their fantasy woman has between a C and a D cup. Again, this is a rather crude measurement, but it at least tells us that guys aren't fantasizing about jumbo boobs; however, they do seem to be picturing something that's larger than average, given that most men selected a choice that was above the midpoint of the scale.

In sum, what all of this tells us is that straight men in America aren't exactly fantasizing about blonde bombshells. Instead, most of them are fantasizing about brunette women of average height who have a normal—but not underweight—BMI, are virtually hair-free, and have an ample bosom.

Who Are Gay and Bisexual People Fantasizing About?

What do the fantasy partners of Americans who are attracted to the same sex look like? And how do they compare to those of their heterosexual counterparts? Let's take a look.

The ladies that lesbian and bisexual women fantasized about weren't that far off from the fantasies of heterosexual men in terms of their body proportions—they were identical in terms of height and pretty similar in terms of weight. The main difference was that lesbian and bisexual women said their fantasy partners weighed about ten pounds more than heterosexual men's ideal. Even so, this means that lesbian and bisexual women are fantasizing about partners who weigh twenty-nine pounds less than the average American woman.

The other characteristics of lesbian and bisexual women's fantasy partners were remarkably similar to those of heterosexual men's, including a strong preference for brunettes over blondes, no body hair, minimal pubic hair (just 2 percent said they fantasize about partners with a full bush), and slightly larger than average breasts.

Likewise, the men that gay and bisexual guys fantasize about share a lot in common with the men in straight women's fantasies. They both picture partners who are a couple inches taller than average and who weigh a bit less than the average guy. However, gay and bisexual men had even stricter standards for weight: their fantasy partners weighed eight pounds less than heterosexual women's. Also, just like straight women, less than one in ten gay and bisexual guys said their fantasy partner is "very muscular"—so, again, the overriding preference is for men who are athletic, not muscle-bound.

As for other body characteristics, gay and bisexual men also expressed a preference for brunettes who manscape. Most reported fantasizing about guys who had at least some body and pubic hair, though compared to straight women, they were more likely to fantasize about completely hairless partners.

Gay and bisexual men's fantasy partners also had above-average penises—7.1 inches in length, to be exact. In addition, while a preference for circumcised penises emerged overall, it wasn't quite as pronounced among gay and bi men as it was among heterosexual women.

In short, what we're seeing here is that, by and large, straight women and gay/bi men have male fantasy partners who are fairly interchangeable—and the same could be said for the female fantasy partners of straight men, lesbians, and bisexual women. The main difference is that, regardless of sexual orientation, men are just a little more demanding when it comes to weight than are women.

The Role of Race in Sexual Fantasy

As you can see, aside from our partner's gender, sexual orientation doesn't play a huge role when it comes to what our fantasy partners look like—but it turns out that our race does.

I found that white people fantasized predominately about other whites. Only about a quarter of them said their fantasy partner was of another race. However, no other racial group showed such a strong same-race preference in their fantasies. For example, Asians predominately fantasized about whites—and this was especially true for straight Asian women and gay Asian men, of whom 75–80 percent said their fantasy partners were white. By contrast, blacks were not fantasizing about whites for the most part (only about one in three were)—but they weren't necessarily fantasizing about other blacks, either. In fact, their fantasy partners were not predominately of a single race. As for Hispanics, they were somewhere in between in terms of their racial preferences, with just over half describing their fantasy partners as white and the remainder reporting a variety of other races. So, like Asians, Hispanics also showed an out-group preference, though it wasn't quite as pronounced.

What all of this suggests is that our racial and cultural background—as well as our beliefs and stereotypes about race more broadly—seem to be baked into our sexual fantasies to some degree. In the United States, whites have historically held the most social and political power, and as a result, they have been the ones who have established the cultural standards when it comes to what is beautiful and sexy. The net effect of this is that it has created a racial hierarchy in the United States when it comes to sex appeal in which whites are at the top and are seen as the most sexually desirable. Within this hierarchy, blacks and Hispanics are somewhere in the middle while Asians are at the bottom. The primary distinction between these groups is that blacks and Hispanics are viewed through a sexualized lens, whereas Asians are not. For example, in the media, blacks and Hispanics are often portrayed as hypersexual or as good lovers. And if they're male, they're stereotyped as having large penises. By contrast, Asians—and especially Asian men—tend to be seen as asexual. Also, Asian guys are stereotyped as having small penises.

My survey results suggest that racial minorities have internalized these stereotypes and this cultural standard of beauty to at least some degree in that—unlike whites—none of them were fantasizing primarily about people of their own race. Asian Americans in particular seem to be most affected by this sex-appeal hierarchy in the sense that they were the least likely to be attracted to persons of their own race and, instead, showed an overwhelming attraction toward whites. This suggests the rather disturbing conclusion that institutionalized racism may carry over into our fantasy worlds in ways that we aren't necessarily consciously aware of.

How Personality, Politics, and Porn Use Shape Our Fantasy Partners

The bodies of the people who appear in our sexual fantasies are also, to some degree, a function of our personalities, political beliefs, and porn-use habits.

In terms of personality, sensation-seeking tendencies play a big role. What we're talking about here are people who enjoy thrilling and risky sexual activities. Sensation seekers require heightened levels of stimulation in order to achieve the same highs that others do, and there's actually a biological reason for this: they have a receptor deficiency in the brain that makes them less responsive to dopamine, a neurotransmitter involved in feelings of pleasure.[6] I found that, regardless of their gender, sensation seekers who are attracted to women fantasize about partners with larger breasts, while sensation seekers who are attracted to men fantasize about partners with bigger penises. The same pattern of associations emerged among people who are erotophilic, meaning they hold very positive attitudes toward sex. So, for people who really like sex and/or need an extra boost of stimulation to get off, bigger breasts and penises are just what the doctor ordered.

Also, for both straight women and gay men, being extraverted—that is, being sociable and outgoing—was linked to fantasies about larger penises. In addition, for straight women only, being neurotic—that is, having more emotional instability—was linked to fantasies about smaller penises. I suspect that both of these associations can be explained by the fact that extraverts are more drawn to sexual novelty, whereas neurotics tend to be put off by novelty. Big penises are indeed a novelty in the sense that most penises tend to fall within a pretty narrow range in terms of size.

Interestingly, Americans' political affiliations also have implications for the body features—particularly the penises—that appear in their fantasies. I found that among men and women, both gay and straight, Republicans were more likely to fantasize about larger penises than Democrats. Why is that? One way to interpret this is that it's simply another extension of Republicans' greater interest in sexual novelties and taboos. However, another possibility is that the penis symbolizes something different for Democrats and Republicans, perhaps that Republicans are more likely to see the penis as a symbol of power or toughness. Then presidential candidate Donald Trump epitomized this idea during one of the televised Republican primary debates in 2016. After being mocked by Senator Marco Rubio for having small hands, Trump replied: "Look at those hands, are they small hands?" After raising his hands for the world to see, he continued: "And, he referred to my hands—'if they're small, something else must be small.' I guarantee you there's no problem. I guarantee."[7] After being elected, Trump reiterated his apparent belief in the importance of size by bragging on Twitter about how his nuclear button is "much bigger & more powerful" than that of Kim Jong Un, the leader of North Korea.[8]

Finally, our porn-use habits are also linked to the bodies that appear in our sexual fantasies. For example, among heterosexual women, those who watched more porn tended to fantasize about male partners with less pubic hair and larger penises. Likewise, among heterosexual men as well as lesbian and bisexual women, those who watched more porn fantasized about female partners with larger breasts. We know there's a major selection effect for body type when it comes to pornography: actresses tend to have larger-than-average busts, actors tend to have bigger-than-average penises, and everyone has far less pubic hair than they do in the real world. My data are consistent with the idea that watching more porn and therefore seeing more breasts and genitals of this kind could potentially shape the type of bodies we find optimally attractive; however, they don't necessarily rule out the possibility that people who are more drawn to big boobs and penises just watch more porn in the first place.

Interestingly, it turned out that gay and bisexual men's porn-use habits had no association with their penis size and pubic hair preferences. This could be because porn use is more ubiquitous among gay and bisexual men and, therefore, has more broadly shaped preferences in this community. This explanation makes sense in light of data suggesting that gay men do use more porn than anyone else, which is thought to be due to the fact that porn is more widely accepted and tolerated in gay men's relationships than it is in heterosexual relationships.[9] At the same time, though, the lack of an association here could also be because gay and bisexual men's genital preferences are being driven by something independent of porn, such as the fact that large genitals were celebrated and sought after in the gay community long before the rise of online porn.

With all of that said, my overall take on the link between porn use and fantasy content is that porn both shapes *and* reflects our fantasies. As direct evidence that porn shapes our fantasies, consider this: when I asked my participants where they think their favorite fantasy of all time comes from, 16 percent said that it directly stemmed from something they saw in porn. It makes sense that this would happen because of something psychologists refer to as the *mere exposure effect*.[10] This is a well-established finding that refers to the idea that the more familiarity we have with something, the more we come to like it—or rather, in the case of porn, the more we like to come to it. Mere exposure doesn't work for everything, though—it only works in cases where our initial reaction is near neutral. So, for example, if you were to watch some type of fetish porn and have a very negative reaction to it, watching it again probably isn't going to make you like it any more. But if it didn't turn you off at first, repeated exposure just might result in more arousal over time.

However, while porn undeniably shapes our fantasies, more often than not it simply reflects our interests, serving as a way for us to vicariously act them out. When I asked my participants whether they had ever searched for porn that depicts their favorite fantasy, fully 81 percent said they had done so. So porn is both a cause of and an outlet for our sexual fantasies—however, it seems to serve the latter role far more often, which makes sense when you consider that most people search for the same thing over and over when it comes to porn. It's only when people happen to start watching a different genre of porn that there's the potential for a new interest to set in—but, again, only if that new genre initially provokes a near-neutral response.

Dream Lover, Come Rescue Me: Who Is It We Actually Fantasize About?

Until this point, we've really only talked about what the bodies of our fantasy partners look like—but who exactly is attached to those bodies? Is it a current partner? A celebrity crush? A comic book hero? Or someone else? Let's take a look.

According to my survey data, if there's one specific person who's likely to appear in your sexual fantasies, it's your current romantic partner. Nine in ten of my participants said they'd fantasized about a current partner before, and just over half (51 percent) said they do this often. No one else comes close. For example, just two-thirds said they had ever fantasized about a celebrity, less than half had fantasized about a specific porn star, and just one in ten had fantasized about a specific politician. What's more, less than 7 percent said they fantasize about celebrities, porn stars, or politicians often. In other words, famous people seem to make pretty infrequent guest appearances in our fantasies.

This tendency to fantasize about romantic partners more than anyone else seems to be true for people of all genders and sexualities, though I found that gay men were a little less likely to say they do this often than everyone else. There's a very good reason why our partners in the real world are our most common partners in fantasy, and it's because our fantasies often include a strong emotional component. The vast majority of both men and women rarely fantasize about emotionless sex. So, most of the time, we aren't envisioning a basic, mechanical sex act; rather, we also fantasize about how we would *feel* during that sex act (e.g., desired, competent, loved). And because it's simply much easier to experience these feelings with someone you know well than with a complete stranger, we disproportionately fantasize about our partners. This rationale helps to explain why I found that women—regardless of sexual orientation—were less likely than men to fantasize about the rich and famous but more likely to fantasize about their current partners. Because women are more likely to have emotion-based fantasies than men, it only makes sense that women's fantasies would focus more on known rather than unknown partners.

With all of that said, when a guest star does make an appearance in our fantasies, who does it tend to be? For straight women, the most fantasized-about celebrities were—in order—Channing Tatum, Ryan Gosling, and Adam Levine. It's not surprising that Tatum topped this list because his body measurements happen to match up almost exactly with what women said they wanted: he's reportedly six foot one and 183 pounds, just one inch taller and one pound heavier than the average fantasy man described by straight women![11] He is literally the ultimate female fantasy come to life.

As for straight men, their most fantasized-about celebrities were—in order—Scarlett Johansson, Jennifer Aniston, and Jennifer Lawrence. Johansson's body dimensions are, not surprisingly, very close to what straight men described as their ideal fantasy partner: she's reportedly five foot three and weighs 126 pounds, two inches shorter and five pounds lighter than the average fantasy woman described by straight guys.[12]

Which celebrities do Americans with same-sex attractions fantasize about? Among lesbian and bi women, Scarlett Johansson came in first. For those who also fantasized about men, Channing Tatum was their preferred partner. Second place on both of these lists went to more androgynous celebs than those straight folks fantasized about: Angelina Jolie and Johnny Depp. Thus, compared to heterosexuals, it seems that lesbian and bisexual women have a bit more of an attraction to people who aren't quite as sex-typed (that is, celebrities who aren't ultrafeminine or ultramasculine).

As for gay and bisexual men, Zac Efron and Jake Gyllenhaal topped the list, with Channing Tatum coming in third. For those who also fantasized about women, Scarlett Johansson placed first. The fact that gay and bisexual men preferred Efron makes sense when you consider that he's a bit shorter and lighter than Tatum, which is in line with the slight differences noted in gay men's and straight women's descriptions of their fantasy man's body proportions. It's also worth noting that Tatum is eight years older than Efron; there's a lot of research out there to suggest that straight women tend to be into guys who are a little older than they are, whereas gay men tend to be into guys who are a little younger.[13] So it's the combination of these minor differences in age and body type preferences that probably account for who came in at the top of the list. However, for the most part, both straight women and gay men mentioned the same names, which means that they largely find the same guys appealing.

Few straight women said they fantasized about specific porn actors, but when they did, James Deen and "I don't know their names" topped the list. Straight women watch the least porn of anyone, and it seems that they're not particularly invested when it comes to who appears on screen. This is likely because, as I've already pointed out, most porn is made by men, for men, so perhaps women just don't find it or the performers all that interesting. By contrast, straight men were much more likely to have fantasies about specific porn stars, and unlike the frequent "I don't know"s written in by straight women, a ton of names were generated by men. However, the three most-mentioned names were Sasha Grey, Gianna Michaels, and Jenna Jameson. It seems that male viewers—primarily straight male viewers— tend to develop more of a connection with or take more of an interest in their favorite porn stars.

Lesbian and bisexual women fantasized about the same female and male porn stars as their heterosexual counterparts, though they generated more porn stars' names than did straight women (probably because they watch more porn). Gay and bisexual men also had no problem generating names of porn stars they'd fantasized about, with the infamous Brent Corrigan being the most commonly mentioned name by far. (Corrigan was underage according to federal law—seventeen—when he began his lengthy career in adult films. He later became so popular that rival filmmakers murdered the director with whom he was contracted so that they could start making movies of their own with him.[14]) Compared to heterosexual guys, bisexual men were more likely to mention names of women who had appeared in dominatrix porn, like Stoya. This is another case where we see sexual minorities taking more of an interest in famous people who aren't quite as sex-typed in terms of their appearance and/ or behavior, which is probably a reflection of the fact that—as discussed previously—nonheterosexuals fantasize more often about gender-bending.

Hardly anyone of any gender or sexual orientation group said they fantasized about politicians, but among those who did— and it was primarily straight people—there was an interesting gender difference: women were far more likely to say they fantasized about Democrats (think former presidents Bill Clinton, Barack Obama, and JFK), while men were far more likely to say they fantasized about Republicans (think Sarah Palin). However, digging a little further into these data, I found that Palin accounted for two-thirds of men's entries, and no other names were mentioned more than a couple of times. So it's not that men are necessarily drawn to Republicans—some straight guys just have a thing for Sarah Palin. Also, it seems that when women are into politicians, they're primarily into presidents, but only the ones who are young and physically attractive (like Obama and JFK) or who have some type of sexual reputation (like Clinton and, again, JFK). So it's not that being a Democrat inherently turns women on—it's just that Democratic presidents to date have tended to have more of the traits that some women find to be arousing than Republican presidents. So that you have some context for these political findings, my data were collected during the second Obama administration.

It's also worth mentioning that the people who appear in our fantasies aren't always real—sometimes, they're fictional characters. For example, many of my participants reported fantasizing about superheroes and comic book characters. Among straight women, Batman was—by far—the most fantasized-about hero. By contrast, Batman held little appeal for gay men, who instead favored Superman and Captain America. I suspect this discrepancy is partially explained by the fact that Batman is portrayed in the comics and movies as more of a womanizer than your typical hero (rumors of a gay relationship with Robin notwithstanding). However, it's probably also due to the fact that he's confident and sexy both in and out of costume, whereas Superman is not. Superman leads more of a double life—he's a completely different person when his alter ego, Clark Kent, emerges. Perhaps that dual identity is something gay men have an easier time relating to, given that many sexual minorities aren't out about their sexuality to everyone in their lives. This reasoning might also explain why gay men were the most likely to fantasize about superheroes in general, given the sheer number of superheroes who have dual identities. As for both straight men and lesbian women, their most fantasized-about heroes were identical: Wonder Woman, Catwoman, and Black Widow. It's no surprise Black Widow was among the most fantasized-about heroines, considering she is played in the movies by the most fantasized-about female celebrity, Scarlett Johansson.

What Do Our Fantasies of the Rich and Famous Say About Us?

Yes, of course, it's titillating to read about the celebrities, porn stars, and superheroes that people want to sleep with—but is there anything we can learn from them? For example, do the celebrities we fantasize about the most—and how often we fantasize about them—say anything about us?

One way to look at the content of our celebrity fantasies is through the lens of our evolutionary history. In fact, Scarlett Johansson and Channing Tatum are precisely the type of people scientists would argue that men and women are evolutionarily hardwired to find sexually irresistible. Let me explain.

Evolutionary psychologists believe that humans have an intrinsic motivation to reproduce and pass their genes along to future generations. To aid our reproductive efforts, nature has programmed us to be attracted to certain physical traits—traits that signify good health and fertility. These preprogrammed attractions are designed to improve our chances of successfully reproducing without our even realizing it.

For men, it is thought that they evolved an attraction to curvy women with hourglass figures because, in study after study, this is the body shape that men are most drawn to. Specifically, when men are asked to rate the attractiveness of women with various body types, the women they find to be optimally attractive have a waist-to-hip ratio of 0.7, meaning their waists are 70 percent the width of their hips.[15] What is Scarlett Johansson's waist-to-hip ratio? You guessed it—almost exactly 0.7.

Being attracted to curvy women is thought to be adaptive in that it increases the odds of producing strong and healthy children. Scientists have found that women who have smaller waists relative to their hips are healthier—not only do they have a lower risk of developing chronic health conditions, but they also live longer. In addition, curvy women are more fertile; research finds that they tend to have more children.[16] In light of this, one way to understand why so many guys are crushing on Scarlett Johansson is that she has precisely the body type that men were designed by evolution to desire.

For women, it is thought that they evolved an attraction to very masculine physical features, including square jaws, lots of muscles, and deep voices—everything that Channing Tatum has in spades. All of these characteristics are the product of exposure to higher levels of testosterone, but the significance of this is that high testosterone is linked to carrying more disease-resistant genes. As a result, women's attraction to "manly" men is thought to be adaptive in that it may help them to conceive children with stronger immune systems—children who will therefore be more likely to survive. This attraction to masculine men is more pronounced in countries with higher mortality rates and lower life expectancies—and the United States, which happens to be one of the least-healthy industrialized nations, is also where we happen to see one of the strongest preferences for masculinity among women.[17]

So, in light of our evolutionary history, the fact that we fantasize about certain celebrities on occasion—and especially celebrities like Scarlett Johansson and Channing Tatum—shouldn't surprise anyone. But let's say you're someone who fantasizes about celebrities or porn stars a lot. Perhaps you fantasize about them far more than anyone else. Well, *frequent* celebrity fantasies are an entirely different matter and shouldn't just be viewed as a simple product of evolution.

For example, I found that people who frequently fantasized about celebrities tended to have a more avoidant attachment style, meaning they had difficulty getting close to others. I also found that people who had these fantasies a lot tended to be less satisfied with their sex lives and relationships (by contrast, those who fantasized more about their romantic partners tended to be more satisfied). So fantasizing about the rich and famous all the time may signify intimacy issues and/or general unhappiness. However, it is not clear whether these fantasies are the cause or the symptom here. On the one hand, it seems plausible that people who are dissatisfied with their sex lives would start fantasizing about people other than their partners. On the other hand, however, it also seems plausible that fantasizing about unattainable people with perfect bodies all the time could lead to dissatisfaction with one's own life and/or reduce intimacy. I suspect that both explanations are true to some extent, but we need more research to know for sure.

Celebrity fantasies don't necessarily always signify trouble on the home front, though. I found that frequent celebrity and porn star fantasies were also linked to having an overactive imagination, sensation-seeking tendencies, and an unrestricted sociosexual orientation. What this means is that, in some cases, celebrity fantasies reflect nothing more than a wandering mind, the search for a little extra excitement, and/or comfort with casual sex. Findings like these are a good reminder that our fantasies—and our fantasy partners—don't always have to have deeper meaning. As Freud is often claimed to have said, "Sometimes a cigar is just a cigar."

How Do We See Ourselves in Our Sexual Fantasies?

At this point, we're going to turn to the subject of how we see ourselves in our sexual fantasies. Regardless of both gender and sexual orientation, almost all of my survey respondents (97–98 percent) said that they appear in their own fantasies at least some of the time. However, it seems that our fantasy selves are not necessarily accurate reflections of reality—and, further, the way we change ourselves in our fantasies depends on both our gender and sexual orientation.

Let's start by looking at how we envision our own bodies in our fantasies. It turns out that most of us have fantasized about having a different body type or shape, but some of us are more likely to do this than others. Whereas about three-quarters of women and gay men had fantasized about changing themselves in this way, fewer straight men (less than two-thirds) had. So straight guys seem to be a little less concerned than everyone else with respect to how their bodies look in their fantasies. I should also mention that, regardless of gender and sexual orientation, the more people said they currently weighed in the real world, the more likely they were to picture having a different body in their fantasies. This isn't surprising, given all of the cultural pressures on us to be thin (if you're female) and fit (if you're male).

As far as genital appearance goes, the vast majority of both gay and straight men had fantasized about changing their penises in some way. By contrast, most women—regardless of sexual orientation—had *not* fantasized about altering their vulvas. So, overall, women were more likely than men to fantasize about changing their bodies, whereas men were more likely than women to fantasize about changing their genitals. This pattern is consistent with the broader cultural messages we hear about men's and women's bodies: there's a lot of pressure on women to be thin, while there's a lot of pressure on men to have a big bulge in their pants. However, it's worth noting that gay men were more concerned about both their bodies *and* their penises compared to straight men, which is probably a reflection of the fact that there's just more social pressure on gay men to have perfect bodies all around.

Beyond changing our bodies, many of us also fantasize about being a different age—namely, being young again. Intuitively, you might guess that women would be far more likely than men to fantasize about their youth. After all, there's a popular stereotype that women are more hung up on their age than men. However, my data reveal precisely the opposite! Regardless of sexual orientation, it's men who are youth obsessed in their fantasies, not women. The majority of both straight and lesbian women I surveyed had *never* fantasized about being younger than they are now. By contrast, most gay and straight men had done so. So why is that? My theory is that it has to do with the fact that men are much more likely than women to regret their previous sexual *inactions*—that is, the sexual opportunities that got away.[18] There's thought to be an evolutionary reason for this: reproduction requires a much lower investment for men than it does for women, given that men's part can be done in just a few minutes. (In fact, the average time from penetration to orgasm for straight men is 5.4 minutes, according to a study in which five hundred guys with stopwatches timed themselves during intercourse.[19]) This means there are more reproductive costs for guys when they pass up potential mating opportunities. In light of this, I suspect that what men are mostly doing in these youthful fantasies is imagining themselves doing things differently in high school or college. For example, perhaps they're thinking about someone they were intensely attracted to but were too scared to approach, and now they're getting a do-over, so to speak. However, another possibility is that women are less likely than men to find their early sexual experiences satisfying and, consequently, tend to reflect upon them less often. This explanation makes sense when you consider that women tend to have their first experiences with orgasm later than men.

That said, while most women didn't report fantasizing about their youth, some women were more likely to do this than others. Specifically, the more that women said they currently weighed, the more likely they were to fantasize about being young again. In this case, I suspect that the focus of these youthful fantasies isn't really so much being younger as it is being thinner.

People don't just fantasize about changing their looks and age, though—they also fantasize about psychological changes. Regardless of gender and sexual orientation, most of my participants had fantasized about altering their personalities in some way. Interestingly, straight men (54 percent) were the least likely to have done this, whereas gay men (70 percent) were the most likely. I suspect this is because, while there's a lot of social pressure on men of all sexualities to be masculine because it is seen as a sexually desirable trait, gay men—on average—tend to be more gender nonconforming in their everyday lives than straight men (though, of course, there is vast individual variability—we're talking only about *average* differences here).[20] As a result, gay men might feel more pressure to change their personalities in their fantasies in order to live up to some perceived masculine sexual ideal.

People can change their personalities in numerous ways, and I did not deeply probe all of the potential traits that people might want to alter about themselves because there are hundreds of ways they might do this. However, one fantasized change that I did explore was being more sexually assertive. To do this, I asked people how often they initiate sex in reality and how often they fantasize about initiating sex. For the most part, people seemed to initiate sex in fantasy as often as they did in reality—this was true for both gay and straight men, as well as lesbians. By contrast, however, straight women—the group that said they were the *least* likely to initiate sex in the real world—were the only group that fantasized about initiating sex far more often than they actually did. This finding makes sense in light of the sexual double standard: in the real world, straight women often fear that they will be judged for being sexually assertive because this isn't a trait that is consistent with the traditional female gender role. As a result, straight women often hold back and let men take the lead. My survey results suggest that women aren't content with this state of affairs and would prefer to initiate sex more often than they actually do.

What Does It Mean If We Change Ourselves in Our Fantasies?

As you can see, whether and how we change ourselves in our sexual fantasies is related to both our gender and sexual orientation—but it's also related to our personalities, our mental health, and how we feel about our current relationships. Before I explain how, I should mention that, in general, fantasies in which we change ourselves are linked to having an overactive imagination, while fantasies specifically about changing our genitals are linked to sensation-seeking tendencies. What this means is that sometimes these changes don't really have a deeper meaning—they just reflect the fact that we like to fantasize a lot or that we have a heightened need for sexual excitement. Again, sometimes a cigar is just a cigar. Most of the time, however, when we change ourselves in our fantasies, it's revealing of an uncomfortable truth—that we aren't happy with ourselves, our relationships, or our sexual desires.

Perhaps not surprisingly, I found that people who had low self-esteem—that is, people who were unhappy with themselves—were more likely to fantasize about changing their bodies and personalities. People who were introverted and neurotic fantasized more about changing themselves as well. Thus, the less confident people are in their appearance and social skills, the more likely they are to fantasize about versions of themselves that correct those perceived deficiencies, perhaps as a way of putting their minds at ease so that they can enjoy a fantasy free of anxiety.

I also found that people who were unhappy in their current relationships, who reported holding less power than their partners, who were dissatisfied with their sex lives or had sexual problems, who weren't having sex very often, who were worried about being abandoned, and who said they have a difficult time getting close to others were more likely to fantasize about changing themselves. What all of this tells us is that, to some extent, changing oneself in a fantasy may signify that one feels inadequate, insecure, or powerless in their relationship. Just like those with low self-esteem, people with relationship insecurity tend to picture themselves in a way that will provide a buffer against further feelings of rejection.

In addition, I found that people who said their favorite fantasy of all time made them feel guilty, ashamed, embarrassed, anxious, or disgusted were more likely to change themselves in their sexual fantasies. This I found to be particularly fascinating because it suggests that when we have qualms about the contents of our sexual fantasies, we change ourselves in a way that will provide some degree of psychological distance. Perhaps if it's not really you—or at least not the current version of you—that's in the fantasy, this reduces feelings of guilt.

This observation ties in with another one of my findings: Republicans and people with religious affiliations were more likely to fantasize about younger versions of themselves. We tend to see our past selves as imperfect compared to the present, so imagining a less perfect version of the self might be one way to increase comfort with fantasizing about sex acts that are threatening to the way we see ourselves now. In other words, maybe envisioning a different version of the self is a way that political and religious conservatives learn to enjoy fantasies about taboo acts with less guilt or anxiety.

In addition to fantasizing about younger versions of the self, Republicans were also more likely to fantasize about changing their genitals, which ties in with our earlier discussion about Republicans being a little more hung up on penis size than Democrats. Whether it's their own or someone else's, Republicans seem to be drawn to bigger penises in their fantasies.

Don't Just Tell Me What You Want, Tell Me *Who* You Want

What I hope you've taken away from this chapter is that when it comes to analyzing the contents of our sexual fantasies, who we fantasize about is just as important as what we fantasize about doing. The people we want as our sexual partners and what their bodies look like say a lot about us—they are products of our evolutionary history and our current cultural context, as well as our individual psychological needs. The way we see ourselves in our sexual fantasies is deeply revealing as well, reflecting how we feel about ourselves, our relationships, and our own desires. Our fantasies are so much more complex than you ever imagined. Every detail—from the activity to the setting to the people involved—is important to consider and may say something unique about us.

Now that we've thoroughly explored the contents of our fantasies and what they mean, let's turn to the link between fantasy and reality. Should our fantasies remain just that—fantasies—or should we share them, maybe even act on them? If so, which ones? And how do we go about doing all of this?

6

Can Science Save Your Sex Life?

The Benefits of Getting in Touch with Your Deepest Sexual Desires

Sexual disorders—including low libido, problems becoming and staying aroused, and difficulty reaching orgasm—are among the most common health issues facing Americans today. Increasingly, we are turning to the pharmaceutical and supplement industries for help managing them because sexual problems are widely seen as having biological causes and, thus, necessitating medicinal fixes. This is why drugs designed to treat sexual problems—like Viagra and Cialis—have become among the best-selling medications on the planet. While these drugs certainly deserve a spot in our treatment arsenal, they are vastly overused. The reality is that most sexual disorders actually have psychological—not physiological—causes. This is hardly a new insight or discovery—rather, it's one that we've consciously chosen to forget because it's an inconvenient truth.

It's just a lot easier to pop a pill once a day than it is to confront and come to terms with sexual repression.

William Masters and Virginia Johnson, the founders of the modern sex therapy movement and the subject of the popular television series *Masters of Sex*, correctly identified psychology as the root of most sexual difficulties back in the 1960s. This is why the therapeutic approach they created revolved around promoting relaxation and building communication and intimacy rather than manipulating people's biology.[1] And do you know what? Their results were wildly successful. The truth of the matter is that most of us don't need drugs to fix our sexual problems, and even if we take them, they're not going to change the underlying issues—like shame, insecurity, and poor communication—that caused those problems to emerge in the first place. If we want to both prevent and resolve our bedroom difficulties, we *must* be willing to do more than take a pill. We have to start getting in touch with—and sharing—our deepest sexual desires.

Express Yourself, Don't Repress Yourself

One of my all-time favorite Madonna songs is her 1995 single "Human Nature," a song you may have forgotten was even part of her catalog because it was only a minor hit, peaking at number forty-six on *Billboard*'s Hot 100. If I had to pick a theme song for this chapter—and maybe even for this book as a whole—"Human Nature" would be it. Why? Because the lyrics unapologetically argue that sex and sexual desire are just a part of, well, human nature. It's not just that, though—the line she repeats most often in this song is, "Express yourself, don't repress yourself." This line perfectly summarizes not just what so many of us are doing wrong in our sex lives but also what we should be doing instead. If you're near your computer, go give it a listen and come back. You'll see what I mean.

When people believe that their sexual desires are uncommon, weird, or abnormal, they tend to repress them—they keep these desires to themselves, with perhaps Google being the only other entity that has any clue. That isn't healthy. When we feel ashamed or guilty about what turns us on, it can potentially lead to sexual performance difficulties. My survey results bear this out. When I asked my participants to rate how they felt about their favorite fantasy of all time, the more negative emotions they reported—things like guilt, shame, embarrassment, fear, anxiety, and disgust—the more sexual problems they had. But that's not all. These emotions also have the potential to interfere with our ability to establish and maintain a healthy sexual relationship. This is because sexual repression leaves us with a lot of emotional baggage and frustration that is all too easy to unfairly take out on a partner. Instead of owning up to the fact that most sexual performance problems stem from our own issues, it's a lot easier to blame a partner for being sexually incompetent. This is a classic ego-protection strategy and something social psychologists refer to as the *self-serving bias*, the general tendency to blame anyone but yourself when you experience failure. As you may have found through personal experience, people don't like it when we incorrectly place the source of blame on them instead of looking inward, another point Madonna epitomizes in a line from "Human Nature": "I'm not your bitch, don't hang your shit on me." It's time for us to start dealing with all of the sexual shit we've been repressing. Stop putting it on your partners or drinking until you forget about it and, instead, deal with it once and for all.

So how do you go about confronting your sexual anxieties? I laid the groundwork for that in the first half of the book by showing you that your sexual desires probably aren't unusual or strange, nor are they necessarily unhealthy. Do you want to experiment with BDSM? Watch your partner have sex with someone else? Do something that's culturally taboo or forbidden? Have gay sex? Sex in public? If so, you should see now that you're totally normal and—in all likelihood—perfectly sane. Odds are that the things you're fantasizing about are the same things that your neighbors, friends, and—I know it's an uncomfortable thought—even your parents are fantasizing about, too. You're not the only one with these desires, so you probably don't have anything to worry about. Stop running from your fantasies and start accepting them as part of who you are.

This means that you need to come to terms with what some psychologists call the *shadow self*, the part of you that consists of all of the desires and urges (both sexual and nonsexual) that scare you because you think you're not supposed to have them. So long as your sexual fantasies remain cordoned off like this, you'll never really feel complete. Instead, you'll constantly be wondering what's wrong with you and how to fix it. However, to the extent that you can begin to see your fantasies as ones that a lot of other people have, too, you can start down the path of self-acceptance. One of the biggest benefits of accepting the fantasies that make up our shadow selves is that it gives us greater control over whether and how we choose to express those desires. As we'll discuss a little later, repressing our desires is how we lose control of them and how our desires begin to control us. I should also mention that just because you acknowledge a fantasy doesn't mean you have to act on it—it's ultimately up to you to live according to your beliefs and values. Recognizing that you have that control is empowering and liberating, and it's a heck of a lot better than spending your life governed by fear.

Tell Your Partner What You Want: The Benefits of Disclosing Your Desires

Self-acceptance is just the first step. The second and even more consequential step, if you really want to improve your sex life, is to think about sharing some of your desires. Undoubtedly, disclosing a sexual desire you've hidden all of your life can be tough. But that's why the first step is so very important—you need to come to terms with your desires so that you can build up the confidence necessary to put yourself in a position of vulnerability. This is probably why social scientists have found that high self-esteem is linked to greater self-disclosure (though this seems to hold true for men more than women, perhaps because self-disclosure might feel especially threatening to men in a culture where they have been conditioned to keep their emotions to themselves).[2] In other words, you need to get good with yourself first before you can feel ready to share something as deeply personal as a sexual fantasy with someone else.

Disclosing your sexual fantasies to a partner has the potential to yield several important benefits. First and most obvious is that if you ever want your fantasy to become a reality, it can't just remain a private mental image—that is, unless your fantasies revolve around something that you—and only you alone—can do. Disclosing your fantasies can do so much more than simply set the stage for you to act out your ultimate sexual desire, though—it just might also improve your relationship, given that self-disclosure has been shown to be one of the most powerful ways of establishing intimacy with a romantic partner.[3] This is because self-disclosure builds trust. When someone reveals a major secret to us, it shows that they're putting a lot of faith in us—and we tend to reciprocate by trusting them right back. If they can trust us to hold their secrets, we can trust them to hold ours.

As those feelings of trust are building, so are feelings of closeness. Through mutual self-disclosure, you come to know someone in a way that most other people don't, which makes the bond you have all the more special. Given these increases in trust and intimacy, it shouldn't be any surprise to hear that research finds that the more couples self-disclose, the happier they are and the more love they feel for one another.[4] Not only that, but high self-disclosers even have longer-lasting relationships! Also, the more that we engage in self-disclosure of a sexual nature, the happier our sex lives tend to be and the fewer problems we experience in the bedroom.[5] Part of the reason for this is that when we disclose our secrets to someone we are romantically interested in, we tend to experience an increase in desire for that person.[6] There seems to be an important connection between our attachment system and our sexual system, which means that self-disclosure and the corresponding feelings of intimacy that arise may be one of the keys to triggering sexual desire. The potential benefits of sexual self-disclosure are borne out in my survey results, too: the participants who shared their favorite fantasies of all time with their partners reported having the most satisfying sex lives, the happiest relationships, and the fewest difficulties with sexual desire, arousal, and orgasm. Of course, there are risks to disclosing one's sexual fantasies, too—and, as we'll discuss below, people sometimes encounter negative reactions that end up harming their relationships. So, while the odds seem to favor positive over negative outcomes, let me be perfectly clear that there are no guarantees here. Great caution and care are therefore essential when it comes to sharing fantasies with a partner.

Believe It or Not, Your Partner Will Probably Be Cool with Your Fantasy

A lack of self-confidence is one of the biggest things holding people back from sharing their sexual fantasies; however, fear about what one's partner will say holds a lot of us back, too. Even though you may be highly self-confident, if you fear your partner will disapprove, you'll probably end up keeping your fantasies to yourself. This makes sense because in order for self-disclosure to enhance intimacy, we need to receive a response that is positive and supportive.[7] When we do not see this kind of response as likely, sharing deeply personal information becomes quite risky.

It therefore makes sense that, among my survey participants who had *not* shared their favorite fantasy with a partner, a majority expected that their partner would respond negatively—especially those whose favorite fantasies involved group sex, BDSM, taboo sex acts, nonmonogamy, homoeroticism, and gender-bending. It's likely that these folks were expecting a negative response because they've been told for so long that these activities are forbidden. After all, they violate cultural norms of gender and monogamy, not to mention the moral prescription that sex should *only* be for reproductive purposes. That said, people don't necessarily expect negative responses to all of their fantasies. For example, among participants who said their favorite fantasy of all time involved novelty or romance, those who hadn't shared these fantasies actually expected that their partner would respond positively. If you think your partner would be cool with your fantasy, then why wouldn't you share it? This is probably a reflection of the fact that so many American couples have great discomfort talking about sex in general, even when it involves things that both partners are likely to enjoy. That's just sad.

If my survey results are any indication, this widespread fear of negative reactions to one's fantasies probably isn't warranted in most cases. When I looked at my participants who had shared their favorite fantasies with a partner, the vast majority reported that their partner had either a neutral or favorable reaction to it. Reports of negative reactions were pretty uncommon. Partner responses certainly varied a bit depending upon the type of fantasy that was shared, though. For instance, with romance, novelty, and BDSM fantasies, 74–82 percent said their partners responded favorably. By contrast, for group sex, nonmonogamy, and taboo fantasies, 65–69 percent said their partners responded positively (note that this does not necessarily mean that the remainder reported negative reactions, given that neutral was also an option). Thus, if you're sharing a romance fantasy, it's more likely that your partner will react positively than if you, say, share a fantasy about having sex with someone else; however, it's worth noting that in all cases, regardless of the type of fantasy disclosed, more participants than not reported that sharing their fantasy was a positive experience that actually improved their relationship.

While it appears more likely than not that a shared fantasy will be warmly received, negative reactions are very much possible. Among those who took my survey, reports of negative responses ranged from 6 percent (for romance fantasies) to 22 percent (for nonmonogamy fantasies). Thus, there are no guarantees that your partner will be receptive to your fantasy, regardless of what it is. Even something like a romance fantasy—which might sound perfectly harmless—could be perceived as threatening to someone if it's presented or viewed as a sign that they are inadequate in some way. You need to think about both how you are presenting your fantasy and how your partner is likely to interpret it. Some clues about your partner's likely response can be gleaned from their personality and sexual history. For instance, let's say your biggest fantasy is to have a threesome. If your partner is low on sensation seeking, strongly believes that sex and emotion go together, is introverted, and is a bit insecure, it's likely that they're not going to be down for experimenting with group sex. However, if your partner is someone who likes to try new things, has enjoyed casual sex in the past, is outgoing, and isn't prone to jealousy, well, they might be really into your fantasy. In fact, they might be into it even more than you! You may find it helpful to reread chapter 4 while keeping in mind what you know about *your partner's* personality and sexual history instead of your own. This will probably give you some helpful insight into which of your fantasies might be a good place to start when it comes to sharing your desires.

Starting a Conversation About Sexual Desire

At this point, you might be wondering how you go about striking up a conversation about sexual desire with a partner. This isn't something that most of us were taught how to do. After all, sexual communication skills aren't usually covered in American sex-education classes. In fact, given the sorry state of sex ed in the United States, I'd say you're lucky if you learned more than just the mechanics of penile-vaginal intercourse! So allow me to offer some tips and pointers that can help to make this process less awkward and your conversation more productive. Before we discuss conversation starters, though, let's cover the basics of communicating about sexual desire.

First and foremost, choose the timing of your sexual self-disclosures wisely and avoid revealing everything all at once. If you overdisclose too early in a relationship, you run the risk of your partner being caught by surprise and feeling as though it's TMI—too much information—and you might scare them off. Self-disclosure, whether of a sexual nature or not, should be thought of as a process that unfolds gradually and requires careful thought with respect to both the timing and setting in which the disclosures occur.[8] Begin slowly, and as you build up mutual trust, the intensity level of your disclosures can increase. For example, if you're a masochist who likes moderate to strong pain, you might start by expressing an interest in light spanking or paddling before busting out the whips and chains, especially if you know your partner is a BDSM novice. Think carefully, too, not just about *what* you're going to disclose but *where* you're going to disclose it. For example, rather than having an intimate discussion about sexual desire while you're out at a restaurant enjoying dinner, aim for someplace more private.

Find a setting that's free of distractions and interruptions, where no one needs to give any thought as to who else might be listening. This will help to put everyone's mind at ease. Even better, aim for a setting where both of you are likely to be in a state of sexual arousal, such as after watching an erotic movie or having a long make-out session. Remember that when people are sexually aroused, their disgust response lessens. So you and your partner will probably be more receptive to each other's fantasies if you share them in a situation where both of you are already kind of horny. It's also worth noting that research has found that we're more likely to self-disclose to a romantic prospect when we're already thinking about sex.[9] Therefore, if both you and your partner have sex on the brain when this conversation starts, the odds are better that you're both going to be willing to share your sexual secrets.

Second, make it clear to your partner why you're sharing your fantasies in the first place. Is it because you just want to learn more about each other, or because you actually want to act these things out? This isn't the kind of thing you want to leave them guessing about. Also, be clear about how and why your partner is a part of your fantasy. Telling your partner that you desire something new or different has the potential to feed feelings of insecurity or jealousy, so try to cut those concerns off at the outset, if at all possible. For example, you might emphasize how your love and trust for your partner makes you want to share things with them that you've never felt comfortable telling anyone else. You might also make it clear how your partner plays an integral role in the activities you fantasize about. In other words, try to validate your partner as you share your fantasies with them, especially if your partner is the insecure type.

Third, keep in mind that as your partner learns about you, you're going to be learning about them. Think of self-disclosure as a transaction—it's something that goes both ways.[10] Through this process, you may discover that you and your partner don't have the exact same set of interests. Don't freak out! This is to be expected. Remember that our personalities and sexual histories say a lot about the kinds of fantasies we're likely to have. So the more different you and your partner are psychologically, the less overlap you're likely to have in terms of your fantasies. This doesn't necessarily mean that you're sexually incompatible, though! Given how common a lot of the fantasies we've discussed in this book are (especially group sex, BDSM, and novelty), it's likely that almost *every* couple is going to have at least some shared interests. And even though you may not share all your fantasies right now, it's possible that you might both eventually grow to want the same things. Remember that our sexual interests aren't set in stone. We can learn new desires as we age and have new experiences, although this is certainly easier if you're someone who doesn't stress out about trying new things.

Finally, think about how you're going to respond to your partner's disclosures. What will you say or do if they express a desire that you don't have or that strikes you as strange or unusual? Think about not just what you're going to say but also what your facial expressions and body language are going to convey. Your goal should be to communicate care and respect both verbally and nonverbally. Projecting these feelings is vital for maintaining trust and eliciting subsequent self-disclosures.[11] If you instead come across as judgmental—for example, if you show a look of disgust on your face, laugh, or say that their desires sound gross—you're going to undermine the faith they've placed in you and call an end to sexual discussion, perhaps permanently. There's a line in Madonna's "Human Nature" where she talks about being punished for sharing her fantasies—you don't want that to happen to you, so don't do it to your partner, either.

Sexual Icebreakers

With that said, let's talk about how to break the ice. Before we do, though, let me reiterate that the setting in which you choose to start sharing your fantasies is an important consideration. Do it someplace private and free of distractions (this means you both probably want to turn your phones off) and, ideally, when you're both likely to be in the mood.

For example, you could have a date night in which you spend the evening exploring some erotic media with your partner. Choose media that you can use as a jumping-off point for a conversation about sexual desire. Depending on your tastes and comfort level, this could be watching a steamy Hollywood film like *9½ Weeks* or *Bound*—or perhaps a movie featuring one of the most-fantasized-about celebrities, like any Marvel movie featuring Black Widow if you're into Scarlett Johansson or *Magic Mike* if you're into Channing Tatum. Alternatively, you might consider reading aloud from an erotic novel (like *Fifty Shades of Grey*), or pulling up a pornographic video you find together online. During or after, you might point out something you thought was arousing ("Wasn't it hot when…") and go from there. This scenario has a couple of benefits. Obviously, one is that sharing this media may put both of you in a sexy mood, but another is that, if the media you select features your fantasy in some way, it allows you to feel your partner out before you lay all of your cards on the table.

Alternatively, you might go to a sex shop with your partner and explore the products on the shelves together. As you walk around the store, maybe you'll even point out and discuss different items that catch your eye ("Ooh, what do you think of that one?"). Not only does this environment have the potential to spark feelings of arousal, but the diversity of products will allow you to gauge your partner's feelings about a wide range of sexual fantasies and activities. You could go a step further, too, and suggest that each of you select a product to try out that night or next weekend.

Yet another possibility is to make an erotic game part of your next date night. Consider this game a type of foreplay, but also an opportunity to share and learn about each other's fantasies. One option is to buy a prepackaged sex game online or in a local sex shop; however, I should warn you that many of those games aren't that great and most aren't focused specifically on fantasy sharing—so if you go that route, do some research, read some reviews, and choose wisely. Alternatively, you might propose playing a game of Truth or Dare or Would You Rather…? These games allow you to save a few bucks, but they also have the added benefit of being endlessly customizable, which means you can add in multiple questions about sexual fantasies and desires.

One final option to consider is to adapt a technique, developed by social psychologist Art Aron, that has been used for decades to build intimacy between strangers in a research lab setting.[12] It involves asking three sets of twelve questions in forty-five minutes. Each set of questions increases in the amount of self-disclosure required (note that you can easily find all of these questions online with a quick search for "36 questions that lead to love"). The first set starts with superficial and factual questions, like which celebrity you'd like to have over for dinner or what superpower you wish you had; however, by the third set they ultimately transition into intense and deeply personal questions, such as sharing your most embarrassing moment. Not only do these questions help people to become fast friends by generating significant closeness in a short amount of time, but they can also plant the seeds of romantic and sexual attraction among strangers (further evidence of the power of self-disclosure!). I suggest taking these questions and swapping in a couple of fantasy-themed questions in the third set, such as: "What is your favorite sexual fantasy?" "What did you fantasize about most recently?" or "If you were creating your bucket list, what's one sexual experience you'd want to be sure to have before you die?" You could also take some questions from the first set and give them a sexy twist, such as asking which superhero they think would be the best at sex and why. This activity could be particularly useful in the early stages of a relationship, not just for getting to know someone more intimately but also for establishing a norm of communication about sexual desire very early on. It could also potentially be helpful for those looking to explore their fantasies with a casual partner.

Regardless of whether you use one of these icebreakers or make up your own, one thing to keep in mind is that discussing sexual desire isn't just a one-time thing in a long-term relationship. Think of this as an ongoing conversation that you and your partner will have at different points over the course of your lives together. Remember that sexual self-disclosure is a process and you want to avoid overdisclosing early on; but in addition to that, keep in mind that your sexual desires—and those of your partner—are likely to change over time. So think about ways to keep the conversation alive. For example, you might do this by subscribing to a "sex toy of the month" club. I mean, who needs a new jelly every month when you could be getting sex toys instead? The nice thing about programs like this is that they create natural and regular opportunities for discussions about sex and trying new things in the bedroom.

One last thing I should mention is that if you're someone who happens to be single and you seem to have a lot of difficulties striking up conversations about sexual desire, you might consider joining a social networking site like FetLife or an online dating service where people specify their sexual interests in their profiles (something that isn't the norm on popular dating apps like Tinder and OkCupid). This not only makes it easier to identify sexually like-minded folks at the outset, but it also removes any potential feelings of awkwardness about discussing sexual desire, because everything is already out in the open.

The Pitfalls and Perils of Sharing Sexual Desires

Although there are a lot of potential benefits to be had by sharing your sexual fantasies with a partner, such as increased trust, intimacy, and sexual satisfaction, be advised that there is no guarantee that things will turn out well. Sharing your fantasies carries with it certain risks. For example, your partner may find your desires to be humorous, disgusting, or scary. And if you end up feeling judged or rejected, there might be deep, long-lasting damage to the relationship. Another possibility is that sharing a fantasy may make your partner feel insecure or threatened, which could lead to a serious relationship conflict or crisis. And then there's the fact that once your fantasies are out there, you no longer have complete control over how that information might be used. It's rare, but people sometimes use their knowledge of others' sexual desires as a weapon, such as by gossiping about it, using it for blackmail, or publicizing it during divorce and child-custody proceedings in order to portray an ex-partner as a "pervert" and, by extension, a risk to the safety of their own children.

Of course, some fantasies are riskier to share than others. However, we do know that people's background and personality traits predispose them to preferences for certain sexual activities. Therefore, if you know your partner well, it means you can probably at least make an educated guess about which fantasies you want to share in order to minimize the chances of a negative outcome. Again, though, be mindful of the fact that there are always risks when disclosing sexual desires. Only you can decide whether the benefits of a given disclosure outweigh the risks and the best way to share your desires with a partner. Be advised that there are no universal rules or principles here; every situation is unique.

So You Shared Your Favorite Fantasy. Now What?

There are at least four potential outcomes that can occur when partners share their sexual fantasies with one another. First, it could turn out that you aren't really into each other's fantasies, but you aren't necessarily bothered by them either. So you simply acknowledge and respect that you're both turned on by different things. If the relationship is on solid footing, the sex is still good, and you're both okay with your fantasies remaining fantasies, then this is hardly a dealbreaker. Nothing will really change, except that perhaps you'll grow closer as a result of sharing something that's deeply personal with someone you trust.

Second, you might discover that you have very different fantasies and this becomes a bone of contention, perhaps because one partner feels threatened or is bothered by the nature of the other's fantasies. At this point, you need to find a way to resolve that conflict. If this happens to you, whatever you do, please do *not* try to coerce a partner who doesn't share your fantasy into acting on it, and definitely don't threaten to leave them if they don't comply with your sexual demands. Attempting to force your sexual will on someone else is *never* okay. With that said, should you find that you and your partner differ with respect to your desired type or amount of sex, you have what's known as a *sexual desire discrepancy*. This is common, and it's something that different couples deal with in very different ways. Some couples find ways to manage it on their own, such as by making a compromise. For instance, two partners who disagree about acting out each other's fantasies might instead agree to simply add some novelty to their sex life in other ways, such as by watching porn together or experimenting with sexy lingerie or sex toys. By contrast, others might agree to open up their relationship, which would allow them the opportunity to find other partners with whom they can act on their fantasies, while still maintaining their primary relationship. For couples who can't find a compromise, couple's therapy may be in order, especially if the desire discrepancy is causing severe distress. If the partners can't compromise and therapy isn't successful, the couple may stay together but remain unhappy, or they may decide to call it quits altogether. Whether a desire discrepancy is worth breaking up over is a decision that only you and your partner can make, but sometimes it's the right call, especially when the alternative involves both of you living in misery for decades.

Third, you might learn that you and your partner have overlapping fantasies, but you mutually decide that you don't want to act on them. For example, perhaps both you and your partner find the prospect of group sex highly arousing, but you decide not to act on that fantasy due to sexual health concerns, like contracting herpes or HPV, or perhaps because you know that you're both the jealous type. Again, nothing really changes in this case; however, you might become closer as a result of sharing your fantasies. In addition, you might potentially discover that hearing your partner describe a fantasy that is very similar to yours is a very erotic experience. Some couples find that verbalizing their fantasies is a major turn-on, and, as such, they do it regularly as a form of dirty talk.

The fourth and final possibility is that you find common ground in your fantasies and decide that you want to take things to the next level: turning one or more of those fantasies into reality. So just how do you go about doing that? For example, if you and your partner want to start swinging, where do you even start? And what kinds of things do you need to keep in mind to ensure that you protect your sexual health and the health of your relationship? Or let's say your biggest fantasy is to explore your masochistic side. What do you need to know to minimize the risk of injury? Uncertainty is one of the biggest things holding people back from acting on their fantasies, which is why I've devoted the next chapter to answering all of your questions about whether and how you might go about turning fantasy into reality. As you'll soon see, just because you want to act on a fantasy doesn't necessarily mean that you should. And in cases where you do decide to go forward, there are several important considerations you should take into account first.

7

Visiting Fantasy Island

How Do You Turn Your Fantasy into Reality?

Let's say you're one of the many Americans who frequently fantasize about, say, group sex. What should you do about this? Should you confine these fantasies to your imagination, or try to make them a reality? If you decide to give it a go, how do you make that happen in a safe way that doesn't end up hurting you, your partner, or your relationship? In this chapter, I will offer a practical, step-by-step guide to making your fantasies a part of your sex life in a way that minimizes the potential risks while maximizing the potential rewards, using insights gleaned from my survey. Along the way, we'll consider how many Americans have acted on their sexual fantasies and what their experiences were like. We will also explore which fantasies tended to turn out the best (and worst) and look at what your personality says about your odds of having a positive experience.

Before we do that, however, we first need to step back and address two very important and fundamental questions. The first is how you decide which fantasies might be appropriate to act on and which ones should never be anything other than figments of your imagination. The truth of the matter is that just because you fantasize about something doesn't necessarily mean it would be a good idea to act on it. Below, I will offer a few guidelines for determining which fantasies are appropriate to consider adding to your sex life and when you might need to seek professional help managing your sexual desires. The second question concerns the potential risks and rewards of acting on a sexual fantasy. If this is something you're thinking about doing, you would be well served by educating yourself about what's on the line here so that you can make an informed decision.

Dangerous Desires: Which Fantasies Shouldn't Be Acted Out?

Rare and uncommon sexual desires tend to be labeled as "strange" or "weird," and for the most part, people think such desires shouldn't be acted upon. Why? Because we, psychologists and psychiatrists included, have long assumed that unusual desires—*all* unusual desires—are signs of mental illness. When someone is seen as having a mental illness, they tend to be stereotyped—incorrectly, I might add—as prone to violence, sexual and otherwise.[1] Therefore, unusual desires are thought to be inherently dangerous and the people who have them are presumed to be in need of therapy. However, this kind of thinking is all wrong.

For one thing, unusual sexual desires are not inherently signs of mental illness. Just because you desire something that's a little different from most people, it doesn't mean there's something wrong upstairs. It doesn't necessarily mean that there's a risk of danger to anyone else, either. The truth of the matter is that most uncommon sexual interests tend to be harmless, such as dressing up like an animal to have sex (or, as it's known colloquially, being a furry). It's also worth pointing out that just because a sexual interest is common doesn't mean it would be healthy to act out. Indeed, there are some very common sexual interests—such as voyeurism, the desire to spy on unsuspecting others while they undress or have sex—that pose a risk of harm to others. What all of this tells us is that we need to stop judging whether sexual desires are healthy or unhealthy based only on how many people in the population have them. Instead, what we really need to do is look at sexual interests on a case-by-case basis and ask ourselves two questions that have nothing to do with how many people have them: (1) Is this sexual activity consensual or nonconsensual? And (2) does it pose an unacceptable risk of harm to one or more people that goes well beyond the usual risks of having sex?

Determining whether consent is present is usually the easier of the two questions to evaluate. Is it clear that everyone wants to participate in the act and is doing so of their own free will? If so, great. Unfortunately, however, consent may not always be obvious, such as in the case of some forced-sex fantasies. As a general rule, it's not advisable to act out any fantasy where explicit consent is lacking. Mutual consent must be clear and unambiguous at the outset, and there also must be a mechanism for consent to be revoked during the act itself, such as a "safe word," in case one partner becomes physically or emotionally uncomfortable.

The "unacceptable risk" question tends to be a bit murkier because different people tolerate different levels of sexual risk. People also have bodily autonomy, the right to choose what they want to do with their own bodies, sexually and otherwise. Therefore, it's hard to draw a neat line here. However, if an activity clearly and significantly elevates the risk of harm during sex, such as extreme BDSM acts that involve cutting or electric shocks, then it's not something I can recommend exploring in good conscience. Of course, what people ultimately decide to do with their bodies is their choice, but it's not my place to encourage folks to act on sex fantasies where serious harm could potentially result.

Allow me to give you a few detailed examples of fantasies where consent is present and the risk is acceptable and fantasies where consent is lacking and/or the level of risk is just too high. First, let's go back to being a furry. This is a quite uncommon sexual interest; just 1 percent of my participants said they fantasized about it often. In case this concept is new to you, what we're talking about here is the desire to have sex while wearing a head-to-toe costume of an animal, mythical creature, maybe even a Pokémon character. I suspect this interest stems, in part, from a desire to temporarily lose one's sense of self, because turning into someone—or something—else can help us to shed our anxieties and insecurities. When you look at it through this lens, it's really not that different from what motivates a lot of BDSM acts. The sex that furries desire is consensual and, aside from the costumes, largely involves pretty conventional sex acts, like oral sex and vaginal intercourse (though it can give the term *doggy style* a whole new meaning!). In other words, everyone who is participating wants to do so, and the activities don't appear to pose a risk of harm that goes beyond the usual risks of being sexually active. So, while the idea of dressing up in a fur costume and getting it on might sound strange to a lot of people, it's really not something we need to be worried about because it checks the boxes of being consensual and not high-risk.

By contrast, if a person's fantasies involve one or more nonconsenting individuals and/or there's a high probability that engaging in the act could result in serious injury or death, this is not something you should act on. These include voyeuristic desires and fantasies about flashing (the nonconsensual kind of exhibitionism). They also include several other desires we haven't yet considered in detail that emerged in my survey, albeit infrequently (no more than 2 percent of participants indicated fantasizing about any of these acts): (1) pedophilia, the desire to have sex with prepubescent children; (2) necrophilia, the desire to have sex with a corpse; (3) frotteurism, the desire to rub up against strangers in crowded public settings, such as on the subway; and (4) "bug chasing" and "gift giving," the desires to intentionally contract and transmit sexually transmitted infections (most commonly HIV), respectively. It should be clear that the reason these interests all fall in the "dangerous desires" category is because they involve a nonconsenting partner (someone who is underage, cannot provide consent, or is not asked for their consent) and/or pose a significant risk to one's own health or the health of others.

If you've fantasized about one of these things before, it doesn't necessarily mean that you have a mental disorder or are in need of therapy, though. My survey results suggest that it's actually not uncommon for people to have very dark or deviant fantasies on rare occasion. Such fantasies sometimes signify nothing more than an overactive imagination—thoughts occasionally pop into our heads seemingly out of nowhere, and they may focus on things we really don't want to think about. If you never have the fantasy again, there's probably nothing to worry about; however, if it happens often and a nonconsensual or extremely risky act becomes your preferred fantasy content, that's another story and an indicator that it's time to seek help.

That said, it's important to highlight that any sexual interest—whether it's common or uncommon, consensual or nonconsensual, high-risk or low-risk—has the potential to become a problem if it ends up taking over someone's life. No matter what the sexual desire is, if it becomes *truly* compulsive in nature, the result can be damaging. Compulsive sexual behaviors are those that people have no control over. To be clear, we're not talking about the people who simply think their behaviors are out of control because they have moral qualms with their sexual desires—instead, we're focusing here on the people who have legitimate difficulties regulating their sexual behavior. Compulsive sexual behaviors are highly distressing to the individual and, when practiced, don't necessarily produce feelings of pleasure or satisfaction. For instance, imagine a man who constantly seeks oral sex partners through Tinder or other hookup apps on his phone at all hours of the day and night. He struggles to control these urges, they're causing problems for him at work because he's distracted, and they're interfering with his ability to establish the kind of romantic relationship he wants. Even though this man has a very common desire that isn't kinky or unusual at all—oral sex—it's still causing problems in his life. This example shows why it's important to avoid drawing sweeping conclusions about whether a given sexual desire is healthy or unhealthy based solely on its popularity. Instead, we need to look at how a given behavior is expressed and what effect it has on people.

Later in this chapter, we're going to focus on tips for turning a fantasy into reality; however, to be perfectly clear, the only kinds of fantasies that you might want to consider acting on are those that are safe, sane, consensual, and legal. Should you have recurrent, intense urges to engage in nonconsensual activities or sex acts that would likely be harmful to you or others, you should not act on them; instead, seek professional help managing your desires. It's also worth seeking professional help if your fantasies—no matter what they are—feel likely they're getting out of control and are creating distress or causing problems in your everyday life.

What Are the Potential Risks and Rewards of Acting on a Sex Fantasy?

Assuming your fantasy is an appropriate one to act on, what do you stand to gain—or lose—by turning that fantasy into reality? A heck of a lot, as it turns out. Let's begin with the possible benefits.

The most obvious potential benefit is that you might enjoy yourself—and I mean really, *really* enjoy yourself. Living out a fantasy can take your arousal to a much higher level than you typically experience during sex, resulting in particularly powerful feelings of pleasure in that moment and perhaps an intense orgasm—maybe even multiple orgasms. (Contrary to popular belief, both men and women are capable of having several orgasms in close succession, though women are more likely to experience this.[2]) And if your fantasy turns out to be everything you hope it to be, or more, it can create useful masturbation fodder for the future.

Beyond sexual enjoyment, enacting a fantasy with a current spouse or partner also has the potential to bring the two of you closer and to improve your relationship. For example, it can help both of you to fend off the Coolidge Effect and, at the same time, fulfill your self-expansion needs (the inborn drive to grow and expand the self). When the novelty of a new relationship has worn off, adding new and exciting elements to your sex life by acting on your fantasies can potentially prevent passion from subsiding and allow it to keep burning. This is precisely what research shows: the couples who engage in the most acts of sexual novelty—we're talking about things like using sex toys, trying new positions, and watching porn together—tend to be the most sexually satisfied and the most successful at keeping passion alive.[3] You don't necessarily need to act out new fantasies every day in order to reap these benefits either—just one shared experience can yield long-term relationship dividends because the ability to recall that experience and reminisce about it can both enhance intimacy and offer a unique way to fan the flames of desire on demand.

Another way acting out fantasies can potentially enhance relationship closeness is through building intimate communication skills and establishing mutual trust and respect. For example, if a couple wants to start experimenting with BDSM, they must not only communicate early and often about their desires and limits but also demonstrate respect for established boundaries. The more practiced partners become at this, the more trust they will place in each other and the easier it will be for them to talk about sex in the future.

Acting on our fantasies doesn't just have the potential to improve our relationships—it also has the potential to resolve sexual problems we might be experiencing, such as difficulties staying aroused or reaching orgasm. How so? The novelty of acting out a fantasy provides a natural way of refocusing your attention during sex away from unwanted thoughts and feelings—it distracts you from what you might otherwise have been thinking about. And if you can lose yourself in the moment, odds are that you'll be better able to maintain arousal and experience orgasm. Consistent with this idea, research has found that people who are into BDSM report less distress and fewer sexual difficulties during BDSM sex than during non-BDSM sex.[4] This suggests that acting on some of our fantasies just might be therapeutic.

To the extent that enacting our fantasies relieves our anxieties and insecurities while simultaneously revving up our libidos with a healthy dose of novelty, our overall health may also stand to benefit. How so? Research has found that frequent sexual activity is linked to a range of positive health outcomes. This makes sense because, after all, sex is a form of exercise: research has found that, on average, young men burn 101 calories during a twenty-five-minute sexual session, whereas young women burn about 69 calories.[5] However, the benefits of sex go well beyond helping us to keep our waistlines trim. Other studies have found that orgasms offer a temporary boost to the immune system.[6] Perhaps this is why those who orgasm the most tend to live the longest.[7] Not only that, but sex might be good for our brains, too: research has found that frequent sexual activity is linked to better memory.[8] To sum it up, if acting on our fantasies helps us to maintain an active sex life, science suggests that this might very well help us to stay healthy and, ultimately, live longer.

One final benefit of acting on our fantasies is that it offers the potential to increase self-understanding. Your fantasies provide the opportunity to fundamentally change the way you think about yourself, including your own gender and sexual identity. There's a lot of social pressure on us to conform to certain gender roles—to dress, behave, and think in ways that are expected for men and women. There's also a lot of pressure on us to adopt easy-to-understand sexual identity labels—like gay or straight—and not deviate from them at all. However, when people act on their fantasies, especially those that focus on gender-bending and sexual flexibility, they are able to free themselves from these constraints. The result can be a very liberating experience that ultimately helps people to get more comfortable in their own skin. Through this process, some may even come to find that other gender labels (e.g., androgynous, genderqueer) and/or sexual labels (e.g., sexually fluid, heteroflexible) are more accurate when it comes to capturing who they are.

At the same time, acting on our fantasies carries major risks. For one thing, it is vital to recognize that no matter how much you try to mentally prepare before acting out a fantasy, you probably won't know exactly how you'll feel about it until you're in the moment. This is because people are notoriously bad at predicting their future emotional states, something psychologists refer to as *affective forecasting*.[9] This means that when you act on a long-desired fantasy, it's quite possible that it could end up feeling more like a living nightmare. For instance, while you might be extremely aroused by the idea of having a threesome with your partner, you may find that actually seeing your partner having sex with someone else makes you intensely jealous: "Does my partner like him more than me?" "Is she going to leave me for that guy?" Because unanticipated and uncomfortable feelings like this might emerge, it is vital to begin by establishing the communication skills necessary to deal with any potential conflicts before going through with your fantasy.

While we have discussed a lot of ways that your relationship stands to benefit from your fantasies, there's also a risk of harm that must be acknowledged. For example, group sex and nonmonogamy scenarios necessarily expose both you and your partner to *relationship alternatives*—other people with whom you could begin a romantic relationship. If one of you isn't very committed to the relationship to begin with, exposure to these alternatives could potentially put you on a path toward breakup.[10] Also, regardless of the type of fantasy you act out, if the experience in general just doesn't go well, there's the potential for reduced closeness and intimacy. For example, research has found that when couples have a BDSM experience that goes poorly—things don't quite go according to plan or someone gets hurt—some partners feel less close afterwards.[11] Again, this speaks to the importance of careful planning and communication.

Moreover, if you and your partner already have serious relationship issues, acting on your fantasies won't necessarily make those issues go away—in fact, it could make things even worse, especially if those relationship difficulties result in a failure to plan and communicate appropriately when enacting a fantasy. If you have fundamental relationship problems, these are probably best addressed through some type of therapy or counseling, because these are not the kinds of things that can be solved simply through exploring your sexual fantasies. You and your partner need to be in a good place and approach your fantasies from a position of strength, not weakness. This is vitally important for increasing the odds of a mutually positive and pleasurable experience.

Aside from the risk of harm to the relationship, there's also a risk to your physical health. Any fantasies that involve new partners pose a risk for contracting sexually transmitted infections (STI) because the more partners you have, the more risk you take on. Those risks can obviously be mitigated to some degree by practicing safe sex, getting tested for STIs, and communicating with your partners about infection status; however, it's important to be mindful of these risks at the outset to ensure you take appropriate precautions. In addition, activities like BDSM—especially acts such as whipping, flogging, gagging, and applying restraints—pose a risk of injury if not performed with the utmost of care. Moreover, extreme BDSM activities have the potential to be lethal, and unfortunately, there are some documented cases of grave injury and death associated with BDSM acts gone awry.[12] Let me be perfectly clear that such outcomes are rare; however, bad things can happen if the partners don't establish clear limits up front, if they engage in activities under the influence of drugs or alcohol, or if they use equipment they aren't familiar with. Even with proper precautions, though, equipment can malfunction (for example, sex toys can break). This means we must recognize that we can't control everything and be prepared to respond quickly if all doesn't go according to plan. In short, there are health risks associated with acting on many of our fantasies, which means safety must be a priority if you choose to make your fantasies a part of your sex life.

Acting on your fantasies may also carry risks for your livelihood and for your reputation. For instance, acting out fantasies about public sex obviously poses a risk of being arrested if others see you, which could possibly lead to fines, jail time, registration as a sex offender, and/or public humiliation, among other things. In light of these potentially serious consequences, I cannot advise or encourage anyone to act on any sexual desire that violates the law.

As another example, if you decide to take photos or videos during sex, there is a risk that your images may inadvertently fall into the wrong hands. For instance, you might get hacked, you might accidentally attach the wrong file to an email or tweet, or (after a messy breakup) your photos or videos could be uploaded to a "revenge porn" website by a former partner who wants to publicly embarrass you.

Obviously, there's a lot to think about here! But, on balance, do the risks tend to outweigh the rewards? In the case of fantasies about illegal acts and activities that pose serious safety concerns, the risks definitely have it. But what about other kinds of fantasies? Could it be the other way around? The experiences of the Americans who took my survey offer some valuable insight. Let's take a peek at how many people said they incorporated their fantasies into their sex lives and how things turned out for them before we ultimately turn to the questions of whether acting on your own fantasies is worth considering and how you might go about it.

How Many Americans Have Acted on Their Fantasies? And, More Importantly, How Did It Go?

The vast majority of my survey respondents (79 percent) said they *want* to act on their favorite fantasy of all time in the future. In other words, for the most part, people want their fantasies— at least their biggest fantasies—to become part of their actual sex lives. But, as you can see, about one in five Americans are content to keep their fantasies in their heads only. This is due, in part, to the fact that 11 percent of my participants described their favorite fantasy as something that would be physically impossible to act out in real life—like becoming another person or being young again—which tells us that a big chunk of the people who don't want to act on their fantasies just couldn't do it no matter how much they might try. So acting on one's fantasies isn't always an option. And even when it is possible, some folks don't want to act on their fantasies for a range of reasons, not the least of which is that acting on certain fantasies could potentially get you in trouble with legal or moral authorities.

However, it's also worth noting that acting on certain types of fantasies—like those that involve forced sex—might not always be safe. Many of my participants with forced-sex fantasies explicitly said they had safety concerns about acting on them. It's important to recognize that when sex is "forced" upon you in a fantasy, you are still in complete control of that situation. A straight female participant in her thirties summed this idea up perfectly: "The fantasy is consensual, because I am imagining exactly what happens to me." However, whenever we act out a fantasy in the real world, we necessarily give up some control to another person—and losing that control can make acting on a forced-sex fantasy risky. This is probably why so many of my participants who had these fantasies reported they did *not* ever want to act them out. Many made a clear distinction between their sexual fantasies and their actual sex lives, such as this female participant in her thirties who identified as lesbian: "While I would never desire this in real life, the fantasy of being taken and ravaged appeals to me." So, with all of that said, it's perfectly okay if you don't want to act on your fantasies regardless of what they are and your reasons; however, it does seem that the vast majority of people want to act on their biggest fantasies if it's theoretically possible—and safe—to do so.

Among those who want to act on their fantasies, surprisingly few have done it before. In fact, less than one in three have made their biggest fantasy a reality, which tells us that most Americans really aren't getting what they want when it comes to sex. What's holding so many of us back? The biggest perceived obstacles are thinking that one's partner would be unwilling or disapproving of the activity, not knowing how to go about it, and being afraid to try it. In other words, lack of knowledge, fear, and communication problems are at the core.

Those of us who haven't acted on our fantasies may be missing out. The overwhelming majority of my participants who acted out their fantasies said that the end result either met or exceeded expectations (86 percent) and, further, that it had a neutral to positive impact on their relationships (91 percent). So, by and large, the outcomes of acting on our fantasies seem to be pretty good. It's also worth mentioning that, compared to those who hadn't acted on their fantasies, those who had reported feeling less guilt, shame, and embarrassment about their sexual desires. This suggests that acting on our fantasies may dramatically change how we feel about them (though it's probably also true that those who feel less guilt and shame about their fantasies in the first place are more inclined to act on them).

But Is This True for All Fantasies?

While the overall pattern described above held when I dug deeper into the data and looked at each of the seven major fantasy themes, I couldn't help but notice that some fantasies were more likely to have been acted upon than others and, further, that some tended to turn out a little better, too.

The types of fantasies Americans were most likely to act on involved BDSM, nonmonogamy, novelty, and passion/romance. Between one-quarter and one-third of my participants with each of these fantasies had acted on them previously. By contrast, the fantasies that were least likely to be acted on were group sex, taboo acts, and gender-bending/sexual flexibility—people were less than half as likely to act on these fantasies compared to the others. These findings are really interesting because they reveal that group sex—the single most popular fantasy in America—is actually one of the least likely fantasies to be acted on. Why is that? In part, this probably reflects the fact that, for people in relationships, it's simply a lot easier to agree on a new toy to try out in bed or perhaps where to go on a romantic getaway than it is to agree on the terms of a threesome or orgy. Finding a third (or fourth or fifth) partner is also just inherently more challenging and intimidating than implementing many other kinds of fantasies. After all, some of us have difficulty finding just one sex partner, let alone assembling a whole group of partners at the same time.

The fantasies people were most likely to act out also happened to be the fantasies that were most likely to meet or exceed expectations. Believe it or not, nonmonogamy fantasies were most likely to meet expectations, with 92 percent of those who had acted on these fantasies saying the outcomes were at least as good or even better than they dreamed! This is likely due to the fact that practicing nonmonogamy is the ultimate solution to dealing with the habituation problem posed by the Coolidge Effect. By contrast, group sex was the least likely fantasy to meet expectations. In fact, group sex was the *only* one of the seven major fantasy themes for which less than half of my participants said the experience turned out better than expected. Also, compared to nonmonogamy fantasies, group-sex fantasies were more than twice as likely to fail to live up to expectations. This probably stems from the fact that most of us don't have a script for group sex. I mean, who does what? With whom? And when? There are a lot of balls in the air, so to speak (sometimes literally). Plus, what happens afterward? Do you just go home? Do you cuddle? Do you stick around for the post-orgy buffet? There can be a bit of uncertainty when it comes to group sex, and that uncertainty sometimes gets in the way of pleasure and creates for a frustrating sexual encounter.

Of course, whether acting on a fantasy meets your expectations isn't the only thing that matters. If you have a long-term partner, there's also the question of how it affects your relationship. Again, the fantasies that were most likely to have been acted out and to have met expectations—BDSM, nonmonogamy, novelty, and passion—were also the ones that people said were most likely to improve their relationships. In fact, between two-thirds and three-quarters of people who had acted on these fantasies said their relationship was the better for it, which makes a lot of sense when you consider that these can all be seen as ways of spicing up a relationship in which the sex has grown somewhat dull or routine.

By contrast, the fantasies that were least likely to help and the most likely to harm a relationship were group sex and gender-bending/sexual flexibility. For the former, I suspect this is just another reflection of the fact that most of us lack a script for group-sex scenarios. For the latter, though, I would argue that this is because American society today still has a lot of hang-ups when it comes to deviations from traditional gender roles and heterosexuality. So, for example, when a married heterosexual woman indulges her husband's cross-dressing fantasy, she might have a hard time seeing him as "manly" afterwards, or perhaps she'll question whether he might be secretly gay. To be clear, he's probably not gay (research has found that the vast majority of cross-dressing men are heterosexual)—but that hasn't stopped numerous women from asking me this question over the years.[13]

With all of that said, my findings suggest that, overall, acting on *any* consensual fantasy appears more likely to help a relationship rather than hurt it. For all seven of the major fantasy themes, a majority or plurality said it improved their relationship, while only a relatively small minority reported harm. So, while certain fantasies—especially group sex—do seem to be somewhat riskier bets when it comes to living up to expectations and improving relationships, acting on any of the seven major types of fantasies seems to have a "happy ending" more often than not.

Is Acting on *My* Fantasy a Good Idea?

Although most people want to act on their favorite fantasies and most who do have positive experiences, this doesn't necessarily mean that everyone should attempt it. In fact, my data suggest that some people may be better equipped to handle the potential risks of certain fantasies than others by virtue of where they are in life and their personality type. Let's take a look at a few of the traits and characteristics that were linked to having better or worse experiences acting on one's sexual fantasies so that you can get some sense of whether you—and your partner—are likely well suited to adding your fantasies to your sex lives.

Are You Happy with Your Current Relationship?

The single factor that was most consistently linked to positive experiences acting on one's fantasies was being involved in a satisfying relationship. Those who had happy relationships reported better experiences enacting a wide range of fantasies, including group sex, BDSM, novelty, nonmonogamy, and passion/romance. The way I interpret these findings is that if you and your partner are going to have a good time acting on your fantasies, you need to start out on solid footing. Of course, there's likely a bidirectional association here: being in a happy relationship probably predisposes people to better fantasy experiences, while acting on a fantasy with a partner further enhances relationship happiness.

It's not just being happy with your relationship that matters but also the way that you tend to approach relationships more generally. Specifically, I found that people who have a more avoidant attachment style—that is, people who have a difficult time getting close to others—tend to have worse experiences acting on certain types of fantasies, especially BDSM and nonmonogamy. This makes sense because these particular fantasies require a lot of intimate communication in order to minimize the risk of someone getting hurt physically or emotionally. Likewise, I found that people who are high in attachment anxiety—that is, people who have serious abandonment issues—reported worse outcomes when it came to acting on a few of their fantasies. For example, they reported less-satisfying experiences with nonmonogamy, perhaps because this scenario is one that can easily feed jealousy and insecurity. At the same time, though, they also reported less-satisfying experiences enacting passion/romance fantasies, which tells us that it might just be really difficult to overpower chronic feelings of insecurity in virtually any sexual scenario. All in all, if you're thinking about acting on a fantasy with a current partner, it's important to be in a relationship where the two of you are close, confident in each other's love, and satisfied.

Do You Feel Good About Yourself?

In addition to feeling good about your relationship, my data indicate that feeling good about yourself is linked to more positive experiences acting on one's fantasies. In particular, I found that higher self-esteem was linked to more enjoyment of group sex and nonmonogamy experiences. In other words, people who were confident in themselves were more likely to enjoy any type of sexual activity involving multiple partners. This may be because higher self-esteem makes it easier to approach the partners that you're most attracted to and/or to communicate your desires to those individuals; however, it may also be because high self-esteem prevents self-defeating or other negative thoughts from entering one's head during sex. Of course, it's likely also the case that having a good experience acting on a fantasy further enhances one's self-esteem.

Related to this, I found that being older was linked to more-positive experiences acting on these same fantasies but also novelty fantasies as well. I take this as another indicator of the importance of self-confidence when it comes to enacting our fantasies. I say this because our feelings of sexual competence tend to increase with age, at least to a point. It often takes a certain amount of sexual experience before people feel like they are good at sex, understand their own bodies, and learn how to cope with their sexual insecurities. This, combined with the fact that we tend to lose many of our sexual inhibitions as we get older (especially when we enter that "zero fucks" stage), suggests that the optimal time to start exploring your sex fantasies probably isn't during your college years but rather once you've built up your sexual self-esteem a bit more.

Do You Have a High Sex Drive or Sensation-Seeking Tendencies?

People with high sex drives reported more positive outcomes when acting on a range of fantasies, including group sex, novelty, and passion/romance. Those with sensation-seeking personalities—that is, a strong need for thrilling and exciting sexual encounters—did so as well. There's a good reason for both of these sets of findings. First, if you're someone with sensation-seeking tendencies, odds are that you'd enjoy acting on your fantasies more than others would, because new experiences are exactly what you require to meet your heightened need for excitement. Second, having a high sex drive means that you'll probably have an easier time staying in the mood during sexual activity. You probably won't be too bothered if a fantasy experience doesn't unfold exactly as you had imagined it, either. By contrast, someone with a lower sex drive needs to keep hitting the right notes and avoid anything that could potentially turn them off; otherwise, their arousal is going to drop pretty quickly. There might be a neurological reason for this, given research that finds people's brains seem to process sexual cues in different ways. By analyzing brain-wave patterns, scientists have found that people who are more sexually active have an equally strong neurological response to both mild and potent sexual cues, whereas those who are less sexually active demonstrate a proportional response (i.e., the stronger the cue, the stronger the response).[14] The implication of this is that if you have a high sex drive, it probably doesn't take as much to keep you stimulated during sex as it would if you had a lower libido. And because our fantasies don't always go according to plan when we act on them—especially group sex, which doesn't have a script—this means that you probably won't have as hard a time enjoying the experience if you're the type of person who is more easily stimulated.

Do You Handle Stressful Situations Well?

One final characteristic linked to people's enjoyment of acting on their sexual fantasies is the personality trait of neuroticism— which, to refresh your memory, is a tendency to have frequent mood swings and to handle stress poorly. What my data reveal is that the more neurotic people are, the less enjoyment they get from acting on their fantasies. Specifically, neurotic folks tend to have worse experiences with group sex, BDSM, nonmonogamy, and passion/romance. All of these fantasies involve doing something new and different—and trying new things in bed (or wherever it is that you like to have sex) can be stressful. For example, research has found that levels of the stress hormone cortisol increase when people are participating in BDSM activities.[15] If you're someone who is highly reactive to stress, then trying new activities like this might not be the best idea.

In sum, what all of this tells us is that the odds that you will have a positive experience acting on your fantasies are higher to the extent that you're someone who happens to be in a good relationship, is self-confident, has a high sex drive and/or a strong need for sexual thrills, and copes well with stress and change. The more of these boxes you check, the better the chances that reality will live up to your fantasy.

A Practical Guide to Enacting Your Sexual Fantasies

Assuming you have a sexual fantasy that is safe, sane, consensual, and legal, you've evaluated and accepted the potential risks and rewards of acting on it, and you've determined that you— and your partner—are in the right headspace to start expanding your sexual horizons, what do you do? How do you actually go about translating your fantasy into reality? In this section, we'll consider some practical tips and guidance that will enhance the odds of having a safe and mutually satisfying experience. These guidelines are expressly designed to counter the biggest things that hold people back from acting on their fantasies in the first place: communication issues, lack of knowledge, and fear. Although no amount of planning and preparation can guarantee that things will turn out well, given all of the variables at play, the following recommendations are likely to help.

1. *Communicate, communicate, communicate.* I can't stress this enough. Tell each other what you want. Talk about your own and your partner's sexual desires in great detail, as well as your limits and boundaries, before taking any action. Of course, you can't plan for everything because unexpected things can (and probably will) happen; however, the less guesswork you leave, the more prepared you'll be to handle the unexpected in a healthy way. Believe it or not, some people (particularly those interested in BDSM) actually go as far as to sign contracts that clearly specify their consent and what their boundaries are before acting on their fantasies. You don't necessarily need to draw up paperwork, though; the key is simply to develop strong communication with your partner and to agree on a set of rules that you will both do your best to respect. Remember: above all, if you're in a relationship, you and your partner need to be in a good place before you start exploring your fantasies together.

2. *Establish a safe word.* No matter what fantasy you're thinking of trying out, you should consider establishing a safe word that you and your partner can invoke should one of you start to feel uncomfortable or wish to leave. Just make sure your safe word is one that's unambiguous and highly unlikely to otherwise emerge in sex—you know, something like *Beetlejuice, Oklahoma, pineapple,* or *lasagna.* (If all four of these words happen to come up regularly when you have sex, well, let's just say that you'd make for a fascinating case report.)

Be very mindful of what using a safe word means—effectively, one of you is revoking your sexual consent. So if your partner utters it during a threesome or BDSM act, it's time to stop, even though you might be enjoying yourself a lot. It's vital that you respect the safe word in the interest of your partner's health and well-being, not to mention the future of your relationship. Actively ignoring a safe word isn't just a major breach of trust, but it can also be a form of sexual abuse. It's also important to keep in mind that some people may find it very hard to utter a safe word, even when they are uncomfortable. Some people just don't feel empowered to do so. As such, it doesn't hurt to check in with your partner verbally from time to time (e.g., "How does this feel?" "Is that good for you?") and attend to their nonverbal signals, such as their facial expressions, to ensure they're still into the activity.

Evidence for the importance of safe words comes from a smaller follow-up survey of sexual fantasies I carried out in which I asked people to tell me in their own words what acting on their fantasies was like. Among those who reported negative experiences, the single biggest complaint was that their partner wasn't as into the activity as they were—and that's precisely why it's important to have an exit strategy in place. At the same time, however, this also suggests that you should really try to turn your fantasy into your partner's fantasy before acting it out. This means working carefully to address your partner's fears and concerns and reducing their uncertainty. Among other things, this means following the next piece of advice.

3. *Before you act, do some research—but make sure you consult reliable sources.* In the interest of both safety and uncertainty reduction, think things through very carefully and research best practices. For example, if you plan to drip hot wax on your partner's body as part of BDSM play, you need to think about what kind of candle you should use and how far it should be from your partner's body to avoid burning him or her. Alternatively, let's say you plan to experiment with nonmonogamy. You first need to think about which form you want it to take. Swinging?

Cuckolding? An open relationship? Next, you need to negotiate the rules so as to minimize conflict and jealousy. There are actually a lot of books, guides, and websites out there with great information on turning your fantasies into reality, such as the book *The Ethical Slut* if you want to learn more about nonmonogamy; however, they aren't all created equal. Ideally, find a research-based source written by an expert in that area, and be sure to stay away from fictionalized fantasy accounts like *Fifty Shades of Grey*, which may be helpful in stimulating sexual arousal but aren't designed to be how-to guides and may contain inaccurate information.

4. *Be safe!* If you and your partner are going to be practicing group sex or nonmonogamy, you'll need to take steps to protect your health by practicing safe sex with each other and with any other partners you might have. Of course, this means using condoms or other barriers, but it also means being willing to disclose instances in which you didn't use condoms and getting tested regularly for STIs. Before you open your relationship, you might also consider getting vaccinated against HPV—a very common STI that is linked to many kinds of cancer, including cancers of the cervix, anus, and throat. This is a particularly good idea if you and your partner are young and/or haven't previously had many sex partners because the odds are better that you haven't been exposed to this virus. And if you're especially concerned about HIV, talk to your doctor about whether pre-exposure prophylaxis (or PrEP, for short) is right for you. PrEP is a daily medication that has been shown to be highly effective at reducing rates of HIV transmission. However, just keep in mind that PrEP isn't a replacement for condoms, given that it only protects against one STI. It's best to think of it as providing backup protection against HIV in case a condom breaks or is used improperly. In short, be sure to think carefully about any and all potential health risks and how you're going to protect yourself—and your partner.

That said, being safe isn't only about using STI-prevention tools like condoms (for vaginal and anal intercourse), dental dams (for oral sex), HPV vaccination, and PrEP—it also means making sure that you approach all sexual activities with care. This means not being drunk or high, to ensure that you and your partner can clearly communicate at all times and don't miss important signals, like safe words. Being sober will also help prevent you from unintentionally blowing past your own limits or attempting a fantasy that you later regret. It's also worth mentioning that alcohol and drugs have the potential to interfere with your ability to stay aroused and reach orgasm, which means these substances could put a serious damper on your ability to enjoy a fantasy experience.

Safety is also about avoiding sexual activities that pose a serious risk of physical harm. For example, extreme BDSM acts (known as *edgeplay*) like strangulation and electric shocks go well past the point of being safe and sane. These are inherently dangerous activities that it would be advisable to avoid. Therefore, you should consider safer alternatives (in this case, milder BDSM acts) that can provide the same sexual thrills you're after. The same goes for fantasies about illegal activities like having sex in public or spying on other people having sex—identify safe alternatives to avoid putting yourself and others in harm's way. Those with exhibitionistic interests or fantasies about public sex, for instance, might find that they can experience a similar sense of novelty and adventure—but without risking arrest and legal consequences—by visiting a swinger's club or attending a sex party. Likewise, those with voyeuristic desires may be able to satisfy their wants safely by joining a legal cam website or visiting strip clubs.

5. *Take baby steps to whips and chains.* When it comes to exploring your fantasies, go slow. Don't jump into intense activities right away, especially if you've never done them before. For instance, a couple

experimenting with bondage might start with one partner simply holding the other's hands above their head or behind their back during sex,
while a couple experimenting with sadomasochism might start with very
light spankings or little bites on the neck. Likewise, if you're interested in
group sex, you might want to start with a group of three before diving
into an orgy or gangbang; alternatively, you and your partner might
test the waters by visiting a sex club or party to simply observe before
you commit to participating in any group activities. Or, if novelty is your
thing, you could begin by purchasing a sex toy or some sexy underwear, you could try role-playing or invent a sex game, or you could
venture out to a burlesque show or strip club with your partner. If you
ease into the fantasy experience, you will either find that it's not your
thing (which is good to know before you get too deep into it!) or that
your inhibitions start to dissipate, thereby allowing your fantasy experience to progress to the point that you can ultimately "give yourself over
to absolute pleasure," if I may borrow a line from one of my favorite
guilty-pleasure movies, *The Rocky Horror Picture Show.*

6. *Remember that what comes after is important.* Acting on a fantasy
can provide a very intense experience for everyone involved. Following such an intense experience, some degree of aftercare might be in
order, during which partners engage in gentle contact like cuddling and
communicate or debrief about the encounter. For intense BDSM acts in
particular, this is often an essential resolution because it provides an
opportunity for reorientation before returning to reality. However, it can
be useful following any shared sexual experiences to check in and see
whether you and your partner felt the same way about it so that you can
adjust and modify your rules and limits going forward, if necessary.

7. *Don't freak out if things don't go according to plan.* Let's say you
don't like the activity as much as you thought you would, or one of you

accidentally crosses a line or breaks a rule. These things don't necessarily mean you have to give up on the fantasy—or your relationship—altogether. Trial and error may be needed in order to fine-tune your sexual likes and dislikes. And if you ultimately decide that acting on this fantasy isn't right for you or your relationship, you can always go back to the way things were before, or consider acting on different fantasies instead. So, for example, trying an open relationship doesn't mean that you have to keep it open forever if the experience doesn't go well—you can go back to being monogamous and try adding novelty to your relationship in ways that don't involve outside partners, such as watching porn together or role-playing.

8. *Remember that keeping passion and romance alive takes work. A lot of work.* Acting out a fantasy with your partner can be a thrilling experience—one that brings you closer and revives feelings of passion for days, weeks, maybe even months afterward. However, to keep those feelings alive for a longer period of time is something that requires sustained effort, a fact that many of us fail to recognize. Far too many people interpret a decrease in passion and romance as a sign that something is wrong with them, their partner, or their relationship. It's probably not. In fact, it's perfectly normal for these feelings to start declining early on in a relationship. Scientists have found that, while sexual satisfaction typically increases during the first year a couple is together, it starts dropping after that in most cases.[16] This happens, in part, because frequency of sex starts to decline. While this may be the normal pattern in the sense that it's what most commonly happens, it's important to remember that passion and romance have the potential to keep going for decades—you just have to be willing to work for it. And regularly sharing and/or acting on your fantasies (something most of us aren't doing) is one of many ways you can potentially maintain an exciting sexual relationship in the long run.

Should You Plan a Trip to Fantasy Island?

I hope you've seen that, when it comes to enacting your sexual
fantasies, the line between fulfilling your wildest dreams and
living a nightmare can be pretty thin. Every fantasy carries with
it a unique set of risks and rewards, and some of us seem to
be better equipped to take on the risks than others. What this
means is that if you're contemplating acting on your fantasies,
it isn't something you should take lightly. While my data suggest
that, more often than not, acting on our fantasies turns out well,
remember that there are no guarantees—and that's because the
outcomes of acting on a given fantasy are determined by the
complex interaction of multiple factors, including the nature of
the sex act itself, the personalities of the participants involved,
and how much communication and planning went into it at
the outset. My advice is therefore *not* that everyone should go
out and immediately act on every fantasy they have. There are
many fantasies that shouldn't be acted upon. Ever. The truth of
the matter is that some fantasies are best kept confined to our
own imaginations, others are best shared but not acted upon,
and yet others we might do well to make a regular part of our
sex lives. Which of your fantasies will take on which of these
roles is something that only you and your partner can decide,
with the caveat that sexual desires that fail to meet the criteria
of safe, sane, consensual, and legal should never make the leap
from fantasy to reality.

While the science of sexual desire tells us that sharing—and
perhaps acting on—some of our sexual fantasies has the potential to benefit us in many ways, enhancing communication about
our deepest desires is just one part of what we need to do if
we want to promote healthier and more satisfying relationships.

There's so much more we can accomplish if we go beyond simply incorporating more of our fantasies into our sex and love lives. As I'll discuss in the next chapter, we need to go further than this and fundamentally change the way that we as a society think about sexual desire, from how we talk to our kids about it to how we treat it under the law. To the extent that we can do this, we all stand to be happier, healthier, and safer in the end.

8

The Path to Healthier Sex and Relationships

How to Break the Barriers That Prevent Us from Communicating About Our Desires

A mericans' marriages are in trouble. Serious trouble.

Of course, we all know that the divorce rate skyrocketed over the last century; however, what most do not realize is that even those who stay married aren't as happy as couples from generations past. In fact, the number of Americans who say they're "very happy" with their marriages declined from 68.8 percent in 1974 to 59.9 percent in 2014.[1] Rates of cheating have been rising at the same time—though, interestingly, only for women. Women's reports of infidelity have increased about 40 percent since the 1970s, whereas men's reports have remained pretty stable.[2] Historically, men have been more likely to cheat than women, but the infidelity gender gap is clearly narrowing. Though we don't know why for sure, I suspect it has something to do with the fact that women's marital happiness has declined more steeply than men's over the last half-century.[3]

211

So what can we do to fix this, to stem this growing tide of unhappy marriages, cheating, and divorce? Undoubtedly, this is a complex question for which there are no easy answers; however, one of the biggest things we can do to promote happier and healthier relationships is to help people better understand their own—and their partners'—sexual desires and learn better sexual communication skills. I say this because research has found that not only are sexual problems the single most common reason that couples enter relationship therapy, but they also consistently top the list when it comes to people's reasons for ending their marriages.[4] The biggest problem areas are sexual incompatibility, such as not agreeing on the amount or type of sex, and infidelity, which is often a symptom of incompatibility in the bedroom.

A sexual disagreement doesn't necessarily have to mean the end of a relationship, though—and this is because, in truth, a lot of the couples who think they're sexually incompatible aren't hopelessly mismatched. After all, my survey results tell us that there are several types of sex fantasies that almost everyone has, such as group sex, BDSM, and novelty. Odds are that most couples have a number of desires in common, but they might not realize it, and sadly, many couples end their relationships before they ever find out because they're too afraid to talk about sex. If these couples instead found a way to begin sharing and, maybe, acting on their sexual desires with one another, they'd likely discover that they're actually pretty damn compatible.

In this chapter, we will explore the steps that we as a society need to take to promote a better understanding of sexual desire and to break down the barriers to talking about our sexual wants and turn-ons. These include reevaluating our approach to sex education, redefining "normal" sex, and changing the way that we approach our relationships. As you'll soon see, by taking these steps, we have the potential not only to enhance our own sex and love lives but also to improve public health at the same time.

First and Foremost, Fight for Comprehensive Sex Education

Sexual communication is a skill that must be learned. However, if we leave it up to everyone to learn it on their own, a lot of people are going to miss out. Formal education is therefore our best bet if we want to help as many people as possible develop the skills they need to establish healthy and satisfying sex lives. But in a nation as politically divided as America, is this kind of sex education even a realistic possibility?

If you follow political news, you might be tempted to think that sex education is a highly partisan issue. After all, Republican administrations tend to funnel federal funds toward abstinence-only programs that stress waiting until marriage to have sex above all else, whereas Democratic administrations tend to funnel money toward comprehensive programs that focus more on teaching students the skills and information they should know if they decide to become sexually active. As it turns out, however, the American public is on the same page about sex education, by and large.

Survey studies of American parents reveal widespread support for comprehensive sex education across the political spectrum. More than 90 percent believe that sex education in middle and high school is important, and further, the vast majority of Republicans *and* Democrats want sex education to cover a wide range of issues, from contraception to sexual orientation to establishing healthy relationships.[5] In other words, there's bipartisan agreement on moving away from the "just say no" approach to sex toward something that teaches students what they want—and need—to know about navigating sexual relationships.

It is imperative that we change our approach, and change it quickly, because by not giving adequate sex education to our kids for far too long, we have allowed online pornography to fill the void and become the default way that adolescents today learn about sex. This is not a model for healthy sexual development because porn sex just isn't the same as real sex. For one thing, in pornographic videos, conversations about sex—including the all-important topics of consent, contraception, condom use, and desire—rarely occur before the action begins. Indeed, it's fair to characterize most pornos as all action, no talk. The idea that communication is completely unnecessary is an extremely problematic message to send a sexually naïve viewer. For another, the sexual encounters on screen frequently offer a misleading view of what good sex is all about—you know, like the idea that the true key to heterosexual women's orgasms is thrusting like a piston. As if that weren't enough, porn stars also tend to have bodies and genitals that are far from average, many of which have been surgically enhanced. This can create unrealistic expectations about what a "normal" body looks like, which probably explains why my survey results revealed that greater porn viewing is linked to more fantasies about partners with unusually large breasts or penises. All in all, in light of the way sex is depicted in porn, we shouldn't be surprised that consumption of sexualized media has been linked to distortions in the way people think about both sex and the human body.[6]

Now, don't get me wrong here—I'm not saying that porn is inherently bad or that we need to get rid of it. That's not my view by any stretch of the imagination. On the contrary, porn can very much be part of a healthy sex life, such as when couples use it together to spark some excitement. Indeed, studies have found that certain types of porn use can actually *improve* people's relationships![7] So, to be perfectly clear, porn is *not* the enemy here. The problem with porn is when it ends up serving as a substitute for sex education, which is precisely what is happening in far too many parts of the United States today.

Many Americans recognize this trend and are disturbed by it, but far too many of them are pointing their fingers at porn and turning it into a scapegoat, labeling it a "public health crisis." Instead, they should be pointing those fingers at our schools—but also at themselves. Schools aren't teaching kids what they need to know and parents aren't picking up the slack, so we shouldn't feign shock and outrage when kids turn to porn as their primary source of sexual information. And we shouldn't blame porn for giving our kids the wrong idea about sex when we don't give them adequate sex ed in the first place. Porn is really only dangerous in the absence of accurate sexual knowledge. We need that knowledge to appropriately contextualize what we're seeing on screen. Think about it this way: if you don't know anything else about sex, it's easy for porn to become your sexual script.

So what does an effective sex-education program look like? Americans would do well to take a cue from the Dutch, who have developed what should be the model for teaching kids about sex throughout the industrialized world. In the Netherlands, rates of sexually transmitted infections, pregnancies, and abortions among teenagers are a tiny fraction of what they are in the United States, and it's because the Dutch are having safer—and smarter—sex, using contraception and condoms at much higher rates.[8] This is due, in large part, to the fact that comprehensive sex education is compulsory throughout the Netherlands, unlike in America, which is covered by a patchwork of laws. This education begins in kindergarten and continues throughout the years with age-appropriate lessons along the way. To be clear, the Dutch aren't teaching kindergarteners the ins and outs of sex (a popular misconception). Instead, young kids spend time learning about their bodies, different types of families, and how to express themselves (so that they can communicate, for example, when they don't want to be touched). As they age, the lessons get more advanced.

The cornerstones of the Dutch approach are understanding and appreciating sexual diversity, learning sexual assertiveness and communication skills, and recognizing that sexual feelings are normal.[9] Specifically, Dutch teens learn about differences in sexual orientation, as well as the fact that penis-in-vagina intercourse is just one way of having sex. For instance, in the most popular sex-education curriculum in the country, Long Live Love, high school students learn that multiple forms of sexual expression exist, including oral sex and mutual masturbation. Students also learn how to stand up for themselves sexually, including how to have difficult conversations, such as when you want to use condoms but your partner doesn't. In addition, students are taught that sexual desire is not something to be ashamed of but rather a normal and healthy part of life. Just imagine if you had been taught all of this in school. You'd probably have a much easier time talking to your partner(s) about sex in general as well as about what specifically turns you on. Having more freedom to explore their sexual desires and less fear of judgment is probably part of why the Netherlands is consistently ranked among the happiest countries in the world.[10] By contrast, the longstanding history of sexual shame and repression in the United States is probably a big part of the reason why Americans consistently report notably lower levels of happiness.

Another important aspect of Dutch sex education is that students have the opportunity to ask questions, and no topic is off-limits. By contrast, in some US states, lawmakers have banned teachers from speaking about certain topics, such as sexual orientation, even when a student inquires about it ("no promo homo" laws, as they're known).[11] Moreover, Dutch teens have a chance to build upon what they learn in school by talking to their parents. In the Netherlands, parents are typically much more open to talking about sex with their kids than they are in America. This means that we can't credit Dutch teens' better sexual health entirely to school-based sex education because they're also in a culture where attitudes about sex are more relaxed and parents play an important role in supplementing what kids are learning about sex in school.

Critics of comprehensive approaches to sex education—like the one Dutch teens receive—tend to argue that these classes will encourage students to become sexually active sooner. However, that's not the case at all. In fact, Dutch teens don't start having sex at younger ages than American teens.[12] So if that's the real fear here, it's totally unfounded. Moreover, comprehensive sex-education programs like this are linked to better sexual-health outcomes across the board than those that emphasize abstinence. In fact, if anything, programs that stress abstinence seem to paradoxically *increase* rates of unprotected sex![13] What all of this tells us is that when it comes to sex education, the more information kids receive, the better—the real danger comes from not providing enough information. A lack of information is what makes our kids vulnerable to the misconceptions about sex and the human body spread by porn—misconceptions that may ultimately be carried over into their relationships to detrimental effect.

A quick point of clarification: "comprehensive" sex education doesn't necessarily have to get into the nitty gritty of *all* sexual desires that people might have, like threesomes, BDSM, and the numerous other interests we explored earlier in this book—those aren't part of any sex-education curriculum for adolescents that I'm aware of, and they don't need to be. These classes don't need to explore each and every possible desire in detail; rather, what's important is that they help students (1) recognize that sexual diversity exists, (2) learn the importance of consent, and (3) build strong communication skills so that they're comfortable having intimate conversations with partners in the future.

We aren't doing our kids any favors when the only thing we teach them about sex is that they should avoid it. The best thing you can do if you're a parent is to ensure that your child receives comprehensive sex education and that he or she feels comfortable talking to you about sex. Not only does this have the potential to improve your child's sexual health, but it also sets them up for a lifetime of success when it comes to sexual and romantic relationships. They will feel more comfortable talking to their partners about sexual desire and pleasure, which has the potential to set the stage for more satisfying, healthier, and longer-lasting relationships down the road.

While supporting comprehensive sex education for adolescents is something that will help our children and future generations immensely when it comes to navigating their sex lives, it obviously won't help those of us who are well past our teenage years. This means we need some adult sex ed, too. Specifically, we need sex ed that can help us to both redefine what we think of as "normal" when it comes to sex and change our script for approaching relationships. To that end, let's take a crash course in sex and love for adults.

Four Essential Lessons in Sex and Love

American adults have a pretty restricted idea of what normal sex is, which is problematic because it leads a lot of people to feel internalized shame about their sexual desires. This, in turn, inhibits sexual communication. Americans haven't figured out how to effectively deal with uncomfortable and unwanted sexual desires either. Our default strategy is repression, which just doesn't work. On top of that, Americans have a very limited and romanticized idea of what a relationship should be, which has the unfortunate effect of setting us up for disappointment and disillusionment time and again. We need a radical change in the way we think about both sex and love, and that's what the lessons in this section are designed to do.

Lesson 1: Relax. Odds Are, Your Sex Life and Your Body Are Perfectly Normal.

People question whether their sex lives and bodies are normal all of the time: "Is it weird to be turned on by this?" "Am I having enough sex?" "Am I masturbating too much?" "Is my penis too small?" All of these concerns are rooted in the same perception problem: we see what other people are doing or we learn about some statistical average, which leads to the realization that we don't quite match up. We then leap to the conclusion that there's something wrong—that we're abnormal. That's a problematic way of thinking that generates a lot of unnecessary anxiety. We need to change our way of thinking and begin to recognize that "normal" isn't just one thing—it's a range.

What we really need to do is start thinking like scientists. Scientists don't look at a statistical average and draw sweeping conclusions. Instead, when a scientist sees an average, the first thought he or she typically has is, "Okay, but what's the standard deviation?" The standard deviation is a separate metric that tells us how spread-out the responses are around the average—in other words, is there a little or a lot of variation? This is a crucial number to look at to establish a normal range around some average. Generally speaking, if you're within two standard deviations either direction, you'd be considered statistically normal, because this is where the vast majority of people fall. Responses that are more than two standard deviations away from the mean are indicators of something relatively rare—something that isn't quite "normal" in that it's statistically uncommon.

To give you an example, let's talk penis size. A review of the penis-size literature that included measurements of over fifteen thousand (!) penises revealed an average erect length of 5.16 inches, with a standard deviation of 0.65 inches.[14] If we calculate two standard deviations beyond the mean in either direction, this gives us 3.86 inches as our lower bound and 6.46 inches as our upper bound. More than 90 percent of the men who were measured were between these numbers, which means that a guy whose penis is anywhere between roughly 4 and 6 inches (give or take a little) is pretty damn normal. It's worth noting that less than 5 percent of these fifteen-thousand-plus men had penises larger than 6.5 inches, which should give you some indication of just how rare a porn-sized penis actually is. And that right there is a prime example of why pornography shouldn't be your barometer for what's normal when it comes to what the human body looks like.

What I hope you see here is that the terms *average* and *normal* do *not* mean the same thing. Stop getting so hung up on whether you're above or below average in terms of your sex life. Relax. Odds are that your sexual interests, the amount of sex you're having, and your genital dimensions are well within the normal range.

Lesson 2: If You're Troubled by Your Sexual Fantasies, Don't Run from Them—That's How We Lose Control of Our Desires. Seek Professional Help Instead.

As I hope you've seen by this point, your sexual fantasies are probably perfectly normal and not a cause for concern. However, should you find yourself fantasizing frequently about something rare or unusual and this bothers you a lot, or should you find that you often fantasize about nonconsensual or risky sex acts, the right way to deal with these desires is not to repress or otherwise run away from them. To do so is to risk losing control of our desires, which could potentially hurt us—and others—in the process.

As we discussed earlier, suppression of unwanted thoughts—whether they are sexual or nonsexual in nature—may be effective in the short term at clearing our minds; however, it's ultimately counterproductive because thought suppression produces a rebound effect, meaning it ironically leads to even more preoccupation with the unwanted thought.

Preoccupation with an urge or desire that you don't want to act upon can be dangerous, especially under times of stress, when our willpower or resolve is weakened. Our ability to exert self-control is a limited resource, meaning we only have so much of it we can use at any given moment, and if we draw on it too heavily in a short period of time, we end up depleted, which makes it more difficult for us to resist urges—both sexual and nonsexual—that we might otherwise want to control. As evidence of this, consider a study in which college student participants and their romantic partners were assigned to a task that either taxed their willpower or not.[15] Specifically, they watched a silent video of someone talking while words appeared at the bottom of the screen. When we see a video like this, our natural tendency is to look at the words because we want to understand what's being said. Half of the participants were therefore told to watch as they normally would (meaning they could look at the words), whereas the other half were told to avoid looking at the words—a directive that required them to exert sustained self-control. Afterward, couples were given a private room in which they were asked to express physical intimacy to whatever degree was mutually desired. What the researchers found was that couples whose willpower had been taxed engaged in more extensive sexual activities, like deep kissing, groping, and removing articles of clothing, than couples who didn't have to exert any extra effort while watching the video.

What these results suggest is that self-control fatigue compromises the ability to resist our sexual urges. Of course, this is not to say that such fatigue necessarily guarantees that we will act on any and all sexual desires we might have, especially those that are unwanted or taboo. In other words, weakened self-control doesn't mean we completely lose the ability to regulate our behavior. However, it does increase the odds that we will give in to the demands of our ids, especially to the extent that there's a combination of the following factors: increased preoccupation with an unwanted desire (stemming from the ironic effects of thought suppression), a prolonged period of stress and fatigue, and failure to plan ahead for how one will avoid acting on unwanted desires when one's resolve is weakened. Of course, some people are naturally more susceptible to these effects than others because not everyone has the same baseline level of self-control. For example, you probably have at least one friend who seems highly self-disciplined most of the time and another who frequently has difficultly resisting temptation. The former will probably have an easier time keeping their sexual desires in check than the latter, regardless of the circumstances.

In short, repression is a maladaptive strategy for dealing with unwanted sexual fantasies. We must instead come to terms with our desires and find effective ways of coping with them, which is where professional counseling and therapy come into play. Such treatment has the potential to help immensely, especially in cases where one has frequent fantasies about nonconsensual or risky sex acts. Unfortunately, however, not everyone who would benefit from professional help managing their desires is willing to seek it, in part because we have actually created some legal roadblocks to seeking help for certain sexual desires, including one of the most dangerous desires: pedophilia. Let me explain.

In many states, psychiatrists and psychologists are required to report to police those adults seeking treatment for pedophilia who admit to having viewed child pornography or who they suspect may have committed any type of child sexual abuse.

Such laws are undoubtedly well-intentioned and were passed in order to hold pedophiles who have acted on their urges accountable in the interest of public safety; however, research has found that when disclosure laws like these are implemented, the number of pedophiles who voluntarily seek treatment to help control their sexual desires drops off dramatically due to fear of potential consequences.[16]

To be sure, there are some pedophiles who want to act on their urges, but there are also some who desperately want to avoid doing so. Mandatory disclosure laws do nothing to detect, stop, or hold accountable the former; however, they discourage the latter from getting the help they want and need, meaning thousands of pedophiles who want treatment and might benefit from it aren't getting it. And when left to manage their sexual urges on their own, many will turn to maladaptive coping strategies like repression, which effectively means we're creating a number of ticking time bombs. Thus, paradoxically, these disclosure laws may actually produce more harm than they prevent.

In short, those who want help managing their sexual desires would do well to be aware that avoidance techniques, like thought suppression, are ineffective and counterproductive. Instead, they should seek professional counseling. At the same time, we must all reconsider whether laws that discourage persons with dangerous desires from voluntarily obtaining help are truly within the best interests of public health and safety.

Lesson 3: Stop Looking for a Soulmate. Instead of Searching for the Right Person, Focus on Being the Right Person.

By and large, Americans believe there's only one person out there for them—a soulmate who is capable of meeting all of their needs, sexual and emotional. Public opinion polls over the last fifteen years or so have consistently found that between two-thirds and three-quarters of Americans believe in this soulmate concept—that there is someone they are *destined* to be with.[17] This belief actually seems to be on the rise, too, with millennials being more likely to endorse it than older generations. The idea of a soulmate is a seductive one. I mean, a relationship in which everything works out easily and not a single need goes unfulfilled—what's not to like? It's no wonder Americans are so drawn to the concept. Unfortunately, however, it's an incredibly destructive one.

For one thing, it sets the bar for relationships and marriages ridiculously high, to the point where we're effectively setting ourselves up for a string of disappointments. Think about it this way: a soulmate is supposed to be the perfect partner. This means your soulmate will be your best friend, a constant source of stability and security in your life, as well as a passionate lover who continually surprises and excites you in the bedroom. Put simply, we're effectively demanding that partners meet two contradictory needs at the same time: stability and surprise. That's a tall order, especially in an era when married couples are spending less time with each other than ever before. (Married couples today have, on average, fifty fewer minutes per day alone with each other than they did in the 1970s.[18]) Is it any wonder, then, that marital happiness is in decline, when we keep asking our partners to do more with less?

Beyond creating unrealistic expectations, the other big problem with the soulmate concept (or holding what social scientists refer to as *destiny beliefs*) is that it changes the way people approach relationship conflict. Specifically, people who hold more

of these destiny beliefs are less likely to actively work on resolving relationship problems.[19] In addition, they tend to break
up faster.[20] People who believe in soulmates are more likely
to bail when they discover that their relationship isn't perfect.
They leave before they've really given their partner a chance
and before making a serious attempt at working through their
issues. Yes, communication and conflict resolution in relationships is undoubtedly hard work, but if you never invest in learning these skills and keep running away instead, you'll probably
never be happy, because relationship conflict is, like death and
taxes, inevitable.

Rather than approaching relationships by thinking that you
need to find the right person, consider the possibility that there
are any number of relationships that could make you happy as
long as you have the right set of skills for navigating them. In
other words, a good relationship is more about *you* being the
right person than anything else. If you think about it, this is
actually an incredibly liberating—and comforting—concept. It
makes the idea of approaching relationships a lot less daunting
because you no longer have to find "the one" amidst a sea of bil-
lions. You just need to find one of your many possible matches.

Lesson 4: Remember That There Isn't Just One Way to Have a Successful Relationship—You Can Chart Your Own Course.

In addition to forgetting the idea that there's only one right person out there for you, you'd also do well to set aside the notion
that there's just one right way to "do" relationships. You need to
cultivate the type of relationship that works well for you—not
the type of relationship that you think you're supposed to have.

Lifelong sexual monogamy is the only model most Americans have for being in a long-term relationship, so that's what they strive for. However, many people find this path to be incredibly difficult, and for good reason: in a romantic relationship, feelings of passion are fleeting. For most of us, passion tends to subside in a matter of months or, if you're lucky, maybe a few years.[21] Many people mistakenly assume that when the passion wanes, it's a sign that the relationship has soured. They come to the conclusion that there must be something wrong if they start finding themselves more sexually attracted to other people than to their own partner. People respond to this realization in different ways; some stay in the relationship but remain unhappy, others turn to infidelity, and yet others jump ship to start new relationships. All of these outcomes leave someone with hurt feelings, but—as I'll explain below—none of them necessarily have to happen. What we're seeing here is simply the Coolidge Effect in action. To grow bored with a sexual routine and be turned on by novelty is to be human.

Now, don't get me wrong. This isn't to say that monogamy is impossible or that it's a lost cause. Monogamy works well for many—and if that's the kind of relationship you want, that's great. However, if you're someone who values monogamy but you also want to keep the passion alive beyond the first few years of your relationship, you need to do something to fight against the Coolidge Effect, such as continually introducing novel sexual activities into your relationship. This could mean watching porn together, joining a "sex toy of the month" club, planning regular date nights, or experimenting with role-playing and sex games. It's worth noting that engaging in novel activities that aren't sexual in nature can potentially help, too. There's a lot of research in social psychology demonstrating that the strong emotions and physiological arousal generated by engaging in new and exciting activities—like riding a roller coaster or white-water rafting—are often mistaken for sexual attraction.[22] What psychologists think is going on here is that when we're breathing heavy and our hearts are racing from a physiologically arousing activity but we're around a sexy person, we have a tendency to attribute our arousal to the person rather than to the situation. So, when we engage in exciting activities, even if they aren't inherently sexual in nature, there's the potential for them to spark sexual interest. In short, it's very much possible to keep passion going in a monogamous relationship if you're willing to work a little and regularly introduce novelty both in and out of the bedroom.

That said, if you have sexual needs that aren't met through shared novel activities with your partner, then you might consider having some type of consensually nonmonogamous relationship. There are a lot of different ways to do this, from swinging to cuckolding to open relationships to polyamory. Different people may be better suited to different styles of nonmonogamy, so you need to figure out what's best for you should you choose this path. For example, if you're comfortable with the idea of having multiple romantic relationships at the same time—relationships in which you're able to meet more than just sexual needs with each partner—then polyamory might be right for you. Alternatively, if you and your partner just want to mix things up every now and then by bringing another person or couple into your bed, then swinging or cuckolding might be the way you decide to go. Or if you and your partner are cool with the idea of going out and doing your own thing sexually, maybe even with a "don't ask, don't tell" rule, then maybe an open relationship is the right option. The key is to figure out what you and your partner are comfortable with and to establish a set of mutually agreed-upon rules and boundaries.

It's worth mentioning that a lot of people are under the impression that couples who open up their relationship in any way must not be in very good situations—that it's a sign of desperation and trouble on the horizon. However, this couldn't be further from the truth. In fact, studies have found that monogamous and consensually nonmonogamous relationships are actually very similar when it comes to relationship quality: nonmonogamous partners tend to be just as satisfied and aren't any more likely to break up.[23] Moreover, and contrary to popular belief, research also suggests that adding an extra partner may actually *enhance* the original relationship. In fact, in a large study of polyamorous individuals a few of my colleagues and I conducted, we found that the more satisfied people were with a secondary relationship, the more committed they were to their primary relationship.[24] The reason for this is likely that nonmonogamous relationships create the opportunity for diversified need fulfillment, meaning that different partners can fulfill different needs rather one partner experiencing pressure to fulfill all of them. Ultimately, this has the potential to reduce relationship conflict—that is, assuming you're not the jealous type. Remember that consensual nonmonogamy isn't right for everyone. In particular, if you're someone who doesn't deal well with stress and/or you have a fear of abandonment or chronic feelings of insecurity, practicing nonmonogamy might increase relationship conflict. This means that when it comes to figuring out what kind of relationship is right for you, you need to know yourself really well first. A great relationship isn't just about knowing someone else really well—it's about knowing yourself and your own limits really well, too.

The key point of all of this is that we need to adapt our relationships to the sexual needs and desires of the individuals involved. In other words, don't get hung up on what you think your relationship "should" look like, but rather negotiate the rules and boundaries for yourself based on your comfort level. No single type of relationship is inherently better than another; different relationship styles work for different people.

Concluding Thoughts: Where Do We Go from Here?

As we established at the beginning of this book, a lot of what Freud had to say about sexual fantasy and desire was wrong. However, he was spot-on about at least one concept, his idea of *polymorphous perversity*. By this, he meant that humans have the potential to obtain sexual gratification from virtually anything. As my fantasy survey revealed, our sexual interests are incredibly wide-ranging. However, whereas Freud viewed sexual fantasizing as a sign of pathology—something that only unhappy people do—my data suggest otherwise. Whether we're happy or unhappy, virtually everyone fantasizes, but who and what we fantasize about—as well as how we see ourselves in our fantasies—can vary considerably from one person to the next as a function of our unique personalities, learned experiences, and psychological needs. Our fantasies are very much a reflection of not just who we are but also where we are in our lives.

By and large, our biggest fantasies tend to reflect our greatest sexual desires, and most people want to make these fantasies a part of their sex lives. As we've seen, however, not all fantasies can or should be acted upon, and it's perfectly fine if you don't want to act on yours—I don't want to give you the impression that you have to be a slave to your own desires. What's most important is that you begin by simply acknowledging your desires instead of running from them. Keep in mind, too, that even if your fantasy is consensual and low-risk and you follow the practical guidelines we discussed for sharing and acting on your fantasies, there is no guarantee that things will turn out well. One must carefully evaluate the potential rewards *and* risks that are at stake and be willing to accept some amount of uncertainty. Remember that when a fantasy escapes the confines of your imagination, it's no longer completely under your control.

That said, sharing and acting on our sexual fantasies has the potential to improve our sex lives and relationships immensely—indeed, the vast majority of Americans I surveyed said that both sharing and acting on their fantasies, no matter what they were fantasizing about, turned out to be at least as good as or better than expected across the board. Thus, there's a lot to potentially be gained by making our fantasies a bigger part of our sex lives.

However, most Americans do not feel empowered to begin exploring their fantasies, and that's something we all need to work on together. We need to break down barriers to sexual communication by tackling shame, insecurity, and lack of knowledge while also changing the way that we approach our relationships, making sure that our expectations are realistic and that we have the flexibility to pursue what it is that we really want. So I'd like to close with a call to action. Here are three things all of us can do that will help tear down the walls that stand between us and our sexual wants:

1. *Pornography is an easy target to blame for almost every sexual problem, but it's not the right one. Don't waste your time and energy fighting the porn industry—fight against poor sex education instead.* As the old saying goes, knowledge is power, and sexual knowledge is no exception. You can never know too much when it comes to sex, and the more you know, the better prepared you'll be to lead a healthy and satisfying sex life. Increasing Americans' sexual knowledge begins with our taking interest in what our kids are learning (or not learning) about sex in school. At the very least, attending to what schools are teaching on this subject will ensure that parents are prepared to fill in the gaps and answer their kids' questions; however, this also provides a valuable opportunity to correct deficiencies in these programs. If you identify problems, you can take those issues to your local school board, which has the power to take corrective action. Remember that most Americans are on the same page about what they want in sex-education courses—but the sorry state of our sex ed isn't going to change unless we actually make our voices heard. And right now, the people most likely to make their voices heard are the minority who support abstinence-only sex education. If we truly want things to change, the majority needs to start standing up for what they believe in.

2. *Stop using other people's sexual desires as weapons against them.* Aside from lack of knowledge, the other major things holding people back from acting on their sexual desires are fear, shame, and embarrassment. People are worried—and rightly so—about how others will react if they share their fantasies. Sharing our desires makes us vul-

nerable. People might laugh or gasp in shock. Or they might use their knowledge of our desires to hurt us, such as by gossiping about them or making them known in a divorce proceeding for revenge purposes. However, if Americans want to start getting what they really want in the bedroom, this kind of sex shaming needs to stop. We'd all do well to recognize that it's actually normal to be a little (or a lot) kinky. Among other things, my survey results revealed that most of us have fantasized about breaking sexual taboos, exploring BDSM, and participating in group sex. Americans have a lot in common when it comes to their sexual fantasies, and we're all kind of kinky in some ways. If my data tell us anything, it's that many—maybe most—of the sexual desires that psychologists have classified as "paraphilic" are anything but unusual to have, at least on occasion. Something that would be unusual would be fantasizing only about that which society tells us we should want when it comes to sex and nothing else. So let's stop the hypocrisy of judging other people for fantasizing about the same things as us. To be human is to be a bit of a freak in the bedroom.

3. *Above all, stop looking for simple answers to complex sexual problems.* Sexual problems aren't easy to solve—in fact, they're incredibly difficult, in part because Americans find it so hard to talk about sex. The result is that we have a tendency to search for simple, easy answers that make us feel like we've done something but that don't actually solve our problems. This kind of approach may even make things worse in the long run. For example, the easy route when it comes to dealing with a dangerous desire like pedophilia involves passing mandatory disclosure laws for therapists. This makes people feel like they've taken an action that will help catch sex offenders and hold them accountable, but in reality, these laws paradoxically may put more children at risk by closing off the only outlet for pedophiles who are voluntarily seeking treatment.

Likewise, many American couples attribute their sexual problems largely if not exclusively to porn. As discussed earlier, porn is always an easy target—and it's a very attractive one, too, because blaming it absolves us of any personal responsibility. However, the reality is that in most cases where porn is viewed as a source of relationship problems, porn use isn't really the issue; instead, it's usually a symptom of something else, such as communication problems, intimacy issues, or a need for novelty that isn't being met. What this means is that blaming porn isn't going to save our relationships and marriages, because if we don't address the fundamental underlying problems, we'll never be happy. We might even see our relationships end before we've really given them a fighting chance, only to start up a new relationship where the same problem inevitably emerges. This is another case where our failure to address the underlying issues ultimately makes things worse in the end and dooms us to repeat the past.

To improve Americans' sexual health and happiness, we need to stop taking the easy way out. The more we rely on simple solutions to complex sexual problems, the less likely we are to experience that happy ending we're all fantasizing about.

Acknowledgments

I would like to express my sincere gratitude to everyone who played a part in turning my long-standing fantasy of writing this book into reality. Thank you to my dedicated agent, Andrew Stuart, for helping me translate my grand vision for this work into something accessible to a mass audience. I also want to thank you for being a tireless champion of the book and never giving up on it. Many thanks to my wonderful editor at Da Capo Press, Dan Ambrosio, for the enormously helpful and clear guidance and suggestions. I also can't begin to tell you how grateful I am for your commitment to letting the science shine through.

Much gratitude also goes to the numerous friends and colleagues who provided valuable advice, feedback, and encouragement at different stages along the way, especially Elisabeth Bernstein, Gurit Birnbaum, Michael Ioerger, Amy Muise, David Ley, Dylan Selterman, and Zhana Vrangalova. I also appreciate the countless conversations I had about this book over cocktails—many, many cocktails—with amazing colleagues from the Society for the Scientific Study of Sexuality and the International Academy of Sex Research. I truly feel like you're part of my family and look forward to our meetings all year.

I am grateful to Janice Kelly for inspiring me to study sex while I was working on my doctorate. Being a teaching assistant for your human sexuality course is what initially opened my eyes to the fact that I could make a career out of studying, teaching, and writing about sex for a living. I truly didn't realize this was even an option before that! My life has never been the same since.

Special thanks to the wonderful team of editors I've worked with at *Playboy*. I'm grateful that you took a chance on me a few years back because the very first article I published with *Playboy*—which just so happened to be about cuckolding fantasies—captured the attention of several literary agents, who said, "Hey, this guy should write a whole book!" And so I did.

Thank you to my parents and siblings for being cool with having a son/brother who writes and talks about sex day in and day out, even at family gatherings. I know you never imagined that this was what I was going to do when I was growing up! Thank you for your support and for being proud of me and my work.

Extra special gratitude and appreciation to my partner in life, Matthew. Thank you for allowing every conversation around the dinner table for the last two years to devolve into some discussion about sexual fantasies. Thank you for your helpful and critical feedback and ideas, the unwavering love and support for nearly two decades (so far!), and the way you encourage me to live my dreams. I couldn't do any of this without you.

Finally, special thanks to the thousands of nameless persons who took my survey and shared some of their deepest secrets and desires with me. Your efforts have made an enormous contribution to our knowledge and understanding of human sexuality—one that will not soon be forgotten.

Notes

Preface

1. Johnson, Z. (2013, October 16). Donald Glover talks *Community* exit, biggest fears: "I'm afraid people hate who I really am." Retrieved from http://www.eonline.com/news/470719/donald-glover-talks-community -exit-biggest-fears-i-m-afraid-people-hate-who-i-really-am

2. Multiple studies have found a link between sexual fantasizing and feelings of guilt, shame, and embarrassment.

   Gil, V. E. (1990). Sexual fantasy experiences and guilt among conservative Christians: An exploratory study. *Journal of Sex Research, 27,* 629–638.

   Cado, S., & Leitenberg, H. (1990). Guilt reactions to sexual fantasies during intercourse. *Archives of Sexual Behavior, 19*(1), 49–63.

3. Freud, S. (1990). Creative writers and day-dreaming (J. Strachey, Trans.). In A. Dickson (Ed.), *Art and Literature* (pp. 129–141). London: Penguin Books.

Introduction

1. According to the Guttmacher Institute, as of 2017, less than half of US states require sex education.

   Guttmacher Institute. (2017, August 1). *Sex and HIV education.* Retrieved from https://www.guttmacher.org/state-policy/explore /sex-and-hiv-education

2. Under the PLISSIT model of sex therapy, the first two steps involve providing clients with permission to engage their desires (as long as they're safe and consensual) and offering sex education that addresses their unique concerns.

Annon, J. S. (1976). The PLISSIT model: A proposed conceptual scheme for the behavioral treatment of sexual problems. *Journal of Sex Education and Therapy*, *2*, 1–15.

3. "[Addyi] was rejected by the FDA once in 2010 and again in 2013, citing ineffectiveness and a too-high risk for side effects.... In clinical trials, somewhere between 9% and 14% of women taking the drug responded to it. And these women had on average an increase of 0.5 to 0.7 'sexually satisfying events' per month compared to placebo."

Walton, A. G. (2015, August 15). Why libido drug Addyi is not the "female Viagra." *Forbes*. Retrieved from https://www.forbes.com /sites/alicegwalton/2015/08/19/fda-approves-addyi-but-it-is-not-the -female-viagra/

4. The National Coalition for Sexual Freedom (https://ncsfreedom.org) has fielded hundreds of requests for resources and referrals in child custody and divorce proceedings from persons who had their sexual desires or practices (most commonly, BDSM and polyamory) held against them.

Chapter 1

1. Freud, S. (1965). *New introductory lectures on psychoanalysis* (J. Strachey, Trans.). Oxford, UK: W. W. Norton.

2. Wegner, D. M., Schneider, D. J., Carter, S. R., & White, T. L. (1987). Paradoxical effects of thought suppression. *Journal of Personality and Social Psychology*, *53*, 5–13.

3. According to the CIA World Factbook, the median age in the United States is 37.9 years old.

Central Intelligence Agency. *The world factbook*. Retrieved from https:// www.cia.gov/library/publications/the-world-factbook/geos/us.html

4. A 2015 YouGov poll featuring a demographically representative US sample found that one-third of young Americans (under age thirty) said that they weren't completely heterosexual.

Moore, P. (2015, August 20). A third of young Americans say they aren't 100% heterosexual. *YouGov*. Retrieved from https://today.yougov.com /news/2015/08/20/third-young-americans-exclusively-heterosexual/

5. According to CDC data, the average age of first vaginal intercourse among both men and women is approximately seventeen. According to the National Survey of Sexual Health and Behavior, most American adults ages eighteen to fifty-nine have sex either a few times per month or a few times per week. According to 2010–2012 data from the General Social Survey, Americans report an average of 11.22 sexual partners since age eighteen.

Centers for Disease Control and Prevention. (2017, August 14). Key statistics from the National Survey of Family Growth. Retrieved from https://www.cdc.gov/nchs/nsfg/key_statistics/s.htm

Herbenick, D., Reece, M., Schick, V., Sanders, S. A., Dodge, B., & Fortenberry, J. D. (2010). Sexual behaviors, relationships, and perceived health status among adult women in the United States: Results from a national probability sample. *Journal of Sexual Medicine, 7*(s5), 277–290.

Reece, M., Herbenick, D., Schick, V., Sanders, S. A., Dodge, B., & Fortenberry, J. D. (2010). Sexual behaviors, relationships, and perceived health among adult men in the United States: Results from a national probability sample. *Journal of Sexual Medicine, 7*(s5), 291–304.

Twenge, J. M., Sherman, R. A., & Wells, B. E. (2015). Changes in American adults' sexual behavior and attitudes, 1972–2012. *Archives of Sexual Behavior, 44*, 2273–2285.

Chapter 2

1. Research on heterosexual college students' attitudes toward and experiences with threesomes indicates that men are much more interested in WWM than MMW scenarios, whereas women show similar interest in both WWM and MMW threesomes.

Thompson, A. E., & Byers, E. S. (2017). Heterosexual young adults' interest, attitudes, and experiences related to mixed-gender, multi-person sex. *Archives of Sexual Behavior, 46*(3), 813–822.

2. Kross, E., Berman, M. G., Mischel, W., Smith, E. E., & Wager, T. D. (2011). Social rejection shares somatosensory representations with physical pain. *Proceedings of the National Academy of Sciences, 108*(15), 6270–6275.

3. For example, the experience of physical pain increases subsequent awareness of taste sensations, thereby making those sensations more intense.

Bastian, B., Jetten, J., & Hornsey, M. J. (2014). Gustatory pleasure and pain: The offset of acute physical pain enhances responsiveness to taste. *Appetite, 72*, 150–155.

4. A large body of social psychological research has found that fear and other strong emotions are often mistaken for sexual feelings. For instance, men walking across a high and shaky suspension bridge are more likely to call a woman they met on that bridge than are men walking across a stable bridge that is close to the ground.

Dutton, D. G., & Aron, A. P. (1974). Some evidence for heightened sexual attraction under conditions of high anxiety. *Journal of Personality and Social Psychology, 30*(4), 510–517.

5. White, G. L., & Kight, T. D. (1984). Misattribution of arousal and attraction: Effects of salience of explanations for arousal. *Journal of Experimental Social Psychology, 20*(1), 55–64.

6. Hatfield, E., & Walster, W. G. (1978). *A new look at love.* Lanham, MD: University Press of America.

7. O'Donohue, W. T., & Geer, J. H. (1985). The habituation of sexual arousal. *Archives of Sexual Behavior, 14*(3), 233–246.

Meuwissen, I., & Over, R. (1990). Habituation and dishabituation of female sexual arousal. *Behaviour Research and Therapy, 28*(3), 217–226.

8. Joseph, P. N., Sharma, R. K., Agarwal, A., & Sirot, L. K. (2015). Men ejaculate larger volumes of semen, more motile sperm, and more quickly when exposed to images of novel women. *Evolutionary Psychological Science, 1*(4), 195–200.

9. Gebhard, P. H., Gagnon, J. H., Pomeroy, W. B., & Christenson, C. V. (1965). *Sex offenders: An analysis of types.* New York: Harper & Row.

10. Pfaus, J. G., Quintana, G. R., Mac Cionnaith, C., & Parada, M. (2016). The whole versus the sum of some of the parts: Toward resolving the apparent controversy of clitoral versus vaginal orgasms. *Socioaffective Neuroscience & Psychology, 6*(1), 32578.

11. A study by Ariely and Loewenstein found that sexual arousal reduces disgust responses in men. A study by Borg and de Jong found similar effects in women.

    Ariely, D., & Loewenstein, G. (2006). The heat of the moment: The effect of sexual arousal on sexual decision making. *Journal of Behavioral Decision Making, 19*(2), 87–98.

    Borg, C., & de Jong, P. J. (2012). Feelings of disgust and disgust-induced avoidance weaken following induced sexual arousal in women. *PLOS ONE, 7*(9), e44111.

12. Gebhard, Gagnon, Pomeroy, & Christenson. *Sex offenders: An analysis of types.*

13. Aron, A., & Aron, E. N. (1986). *Love and the expansion of self: Understanding attraction and satisfaction.* New York: Hemisphere.

14. Baumeister, R. F., & Leary, M. R. (1995). The need to belong: Desire for interpersonal attachments as a fundamental human motivation. *Psychological Bulletin, 117*(3), 497–529.

15. Lawrence, A. A. (2017). Autogynephilia and the typology of male-to-female transsexualism. *European Psychologist, 22,* 39–54.

16. Ogas, O., & Gaddam, S. (2011). *A billion wicked thoughts: What the internet tells us about sexual relationships.* London: Penguin.

Chapter 3

1. LeVay, S. (2016). *Gay, straight, and the reason why: The science of sexual orientation.* Oxford, UK: Oxford University Press.

2. Bicks, J. (Writer), & Thomas, P. (Director). (2000). Boy, girl, boy, girl… [Television series episode]. In Star, D. (Executive Producer), *Sex and the City.* Beverly Hills, CA: Darren Star Productions.

3. Chivers, M. L., Rieger, G., Latty, E., & Bailey, J. M. (2004). A sex difference in the specificity of sexual arousal. *Psychological Science, 15*(11), 736–744.

4. Adams, H. E., Wright, L. W., & Lohr, B. A. (1996). Is homophobia associated with homosexual arousal? *Journal of Abnormal Psychology, 105*(3), 440–445.

5. Baumeister, R. F. (2000). Gender differences in erotic plasticity: The female sex drive as socially flexible and responsive. *Psychological Bulletin, 126*(3), 347–374.

6. Chivers, Rieger, Latty, & Bailey. A sex difference in the specificity of sexual arousal.

7. Kuhle, B. X., & Radtke, S. (2013). Born both ways: The alloparenting hypothesis for sexual fluidity in women. *Evolutionary Psychology, 11*(2), 304–323.

8. Baumeister. Gender differences in erotic plasticity.

9. Ellis, B. J., & Symons, D. (1990). Sex differences in sexual fantasy: An evolutionary psychological approach. *Journal of Sex Research, 27,* 527–555.

10. On opening weekend, the audience for *Fifty Shades of Grey* was 68 percent female.

    Lang, B. (2015, February 15). Box office: "Fifty Shades of Grey" explodes with record-breaking $81.7 million. *Variety.* Retrieved from http://variety.com/2015/film/box-office/box-office-fifty-shades-of-grey-explodes-with-record-breaking-81-7-million-1201434486/

11. Baumeister, R. F. (2014). *Masochism and the self.* New York: Psychology Press.

12. Kilgallon, S. J., & Simmons, L. W. (2005). Image content influences men's semen quality. *Biology Letters, 22,* 253–255.

13. Gallup, G. G., Burch, R. L., Zappieri, M. L., Parvez, R. A., Stockwell, M. L., & Davis, J. A. (2003). The human penis as a semen displacement device. *Evolution and Human Behavior, 24,* 277–289.

14. Gallup, Burch, Zappieri, Parvez, Stockwell, & Davis. The human penis as a semen displacement device.

15. Dawson, S. J., Bannerman, B. A., & Lalumière, M. L. (2016). Paraphilic interests: An examination of sex differences in a nonclinical sample. *Sexual Abuse, 28*(1), 20–45.

16. Byrnes, J. P., Miller, D. C., & Schafer, W. D. (1999). Gender differences in risk taking: A meta-analysis. *Psychological Bulletin, 125*(3), 367–383.

17. Dawson, Bannerman, & Lalumière. Paraphilic interests.

18. Grubbs, J. B., Exline, J. J., Pargament, K. I., Hook, J. N., & Carlisle, R. D. (2015). Transgression as addiction: Religiosity and moral disapproval as predictors of perceived addiction to pornography. *Archives of Sexual Behavior, 44*(1), 125–136.

19. Blanchard, R., & Collins, P. I. (1993). Men with sexual interest in transvestites, transsexuals, and she-males. *Journal of Nervous and Mental Disease, 181*(9), 570–575; Hsu, K. J., Rosenthal, A. M., Miller, D. I., & Bailey, J. M. (2016). Who are gynandromorphophilic men? Characterizing men with sexual interest in transgender women. *Psychological Medicine, 46*(4), 819–827.

20. Ogas, O., & Gaddam, S. (2011). *A billion wicked thoughts: What the internet tells us about sexual relationships.* London: Penguin.

21. Blanchard, R. (1993). Varieties of autogynephilia and their relationship to gender dysphoria. *Archives of Sexual Behavior, 22*(3), 241–251.

22. Cameron, L. (2013, April 11). How the psychiatrist who co-wrote the manual on sex talks about sex. *Motherboard.* Retrieved from https://motherboard.vice.com/en_us/article/ypp93m/heres-how-the-guy-who-wrote-the-manual-on-sex-talks-about-sex

23. In a study of 232 male-to-female transsexuals followed for a year after surgery, "participants reported overwhelmingly that they were happy with their SRS [sex reassignment surgery] results and that SRS had greatly improved the quality of their lives. None reported outright regret and only a few expressed even occasional regret."

    Lawrence, A. A. (2003). Factors associated with satisfaction or regret following male-to-female sex reassignment surgery. *Archives of Sexual Behavior, 32*(4), 299–315.

Chapter 4

1. Brehm, J. W. (1966). *A theory of psychological reactance.* Oxford, UK: Academic Press.

2. Haldeman, D. C. (2002). Gay rights, patient rights: The implications of sexual orientation conversion therapy. *Professional Psychology: Research and Practice, 33*(3), 260–264.

3. Hatemi, P. K., Crabtree, C., & McDermott, R. (2017). The relationship between sexual preferences and political orientations: Do positions in the bedroom affect positions in the ballot box? *Personality and Individual Differences, 105*, 318–325.

4. Smith, C. V., & Shaffer, M. J. (2013). Gone but not forgotten: Virginity loss and current sexual satisfaction. *Journal of Sex & Marital Therapy, 39*(2), 96–111.

5. A 2011 survey of 1,018 American adults found that one in ten men and one in four women reported having been sexually harassed in the workplace.

   ABC News / Washington Post. (2011, November 16). *One in four U.S. women reports workplace harassment* [Press release]. Retrieved from http://www.langerresearch.com/wp-content/uploads/1130a2 WorkplaceHarassment.pdf

6. Richters, J., De Visser, R. O., Rissel, C. E., Grulich, A. E., & Smith, A. (2008). Demographic and psychosocial features of participants in bondage and discipline, "sadomasochism" or dominance and submission (BDSM): Data from a national survey. *Journal of Sexual Medicine, 5*(7), 1660–1668.

7. Devor, H. (1994). Transsexualism, dissociation, and child abuse: An initial discussion based on nonclinical data. *Journal of Psychology & Human Sexuality, 6*(3), 49–72; Dulcan, M. K., & Lee, P. A. (1984). Transsexualism in the adolescent girl. *Journal of the American Academy of Child Psychiatry, 23*(3), 354–361.

8. Bradford, J. M. W. (1999). The paraphilias, obsessive-compulsive spectrum disorder, and the treatment of sexually deviant behavior. *Psychiatric Quarterly, 70*, 209–219.

9. Perera, H., Gadambanathan, T., & Weerasiri, S., (2011). Gender identity disorder presenting in a girl with Asperger's disorder and obsessive compulsive disorder. *Ceylon Medical Journal, 48*(2), 57–58; Safer, D. L., Bullock, K. D., & Safer, J. D. (2016). Obsessive-compulsive disorder presenting as gender dysphoria/gender incongruence: A case report and literature review. *AACE Clinical Case Reports, 2*(3), e268–e271.

10. Wismeijer, A. A., & Assen, M. A. (2013). Psychological character-
    istics of BDSM practitioners. *Journal of Sexual Medicine, 10*(8),
    1943–1952.

11. Allen, D. J., & Oleson, T. (1999). Shame and internalized homophobia
    in gay men. *Journal of Homosexuality, 37*(3), 33–43.

Chapter 5

1. Fryar, C. D., Gu, Q., Ogden, C. L., & Flegal, K. (2016, August). *Anthropometric reference data for children and adults: United States,
   2011–2014.* Centers for Disease Control and Prevention, National
   Center for Health Statistics. Vital and Health Statistics Series 3, No. 39.
   Retrieved from https://www.cdc.gov/nchs/data/series/sr_03/sr03_039.pdf

2. Fryar, Gu, Ogden, & Flegal. *Anthropometric reference data for children and adults.*

3. Veale, D., Miles, S., Bramley, S., Muir, G., & Hodsoll, J. (2015). Am
   I normal? A systematic review and construction of nomograms for
   flaccid and erect penis length and circumference in up to 15,521 men.
   BJU International, 115(6), 978–986.

4. Prause, N., Park, J., Leung, S., & Miller, G. (2015). Women's preferences for penis size: A new research method using selection among
   3D models. *PLOS ONE, 10*(9), e0133079.

5. Heights and weights of models. UCLA College Statistics. (2002).
   Retrieved from http://www.stat.ucla.edu/~vlew/stat10/archival/fa02
   /handouts/modeling.pdf

6. Campbell, B. C., Dreber, A., Apicella, C. L., Eisenberg, D. T., Gray, P.
   B., Little, A. C., ... Lum, J. K. (2010). Testosterone exposure, dopami-
   nergic reward, and sensation-seeking in young men. *Physiology &
   Behavior, 99*(4), 451–456.

7. Krieg, G. (2016, March 4). Donald Trump defends size of penis. *CNN.*
   Retrieved from http://www.cnn.com/2016/03/03/politics/donald
   -trump-small-hands-marco-rubio/index.html

8. Carter, B. (2018, January 2). Social media mocks Trump for bragging
   about the size of his nuclear button. *The Hill.* Retrieved from http://

thehill.com/blogs/blog-briefing-room/news/367160-social-media
-mocks-trump-for-bragging-about-the-size-of-his

9. Hald, G. M., & Štulhofer, A. (2016). What types of pornography do people use and do they cluster? Assessing types and categories of pornography consumption in a large-scale online sample. *Journal of Sex Research, 53*(7), 849–859.

10. Zajonc, R. B. (2001). Mere exposure: A gateway to the subliminal. *Current Directions in Psychological Science, 10*(6), 224–228.

11. Channing Tatum height and weight: measurements. (n.d.) *Celebrity Height and Weight.* Retrieved from http://heightandweights .com/channing-tatum/

12. Scarlett Johansson body measurements. (n.d.) *Celebrity Inside.* Retrieved from http://celebrityinside.com/body-measurements/ actress/scarlett-johansson-body-measurements-height-weight-shoe -bra-size-stats/

13. Antfolk, J. (2017). Age limits: Men's and women's youngest and oldest considered and actual sex partners. *Evolutionary Psychology, 15*(1), 1–9.

14. Tan, N. (2016, May 13). The real "King Cobra" killer speaks out from prison, shares his thoughts on James Franco's film. *Gay Star News.* Retrieved from https://www.gaystarnews.com/article/king-cobra -prison-joseph-kerekes/#gs.Bq06CoU

15. Singh, D., Dixson, B. J., Jessop, T. S., Morgan, B., & Dixson, A. F. (2010). Cross-cultural consensus for waist-hip ratio and women's attractiveness. *Evolution and Human Behavior, 31*(3), 176–181.

16. Butovskaya, M., Sorokowska, A., Karwowski, M., Sabiniewicz, A., Fedenok, J., Dronova, D.,…Sorokowski, P. (2017). Waist-to-hip ratio, body-mass index, age and number of children in seven traditional societies. *Scientific Reports, 7.*

17. DeBruine, L. M., Jones, B. C., Crawford, J. R., Welling, L. L. M., & Little, A. C. (2010). The health of a nation predicts their mate preferences: Cross-cultural variation in women's preferences for masculinized male faces. *Proceedings of the Royal Society B, 277*(1692), 2405–2410. doi:10.1098/rspb.2009.2184

18. Galperin, A., Haselton, M. G., Frederick, D. A., Poore, J., von Hippel, W., Buss, D. M., & Gonzaga, G. C. (2013). Sexual regret: Evidence for evolved sex differences. *Archives of Sexual Behavior, 42*(7), 1145–1161.

19. Waldinger, M. D., Quinn, P., Dilleen, M., Mundayat, R., Schweitzer, D. H., & Boolell, M. (2005). Ejaculation disorders: A multinational population survey of intravaginal ejaculation latency time. *Journal of Sexual Medicine, 2*(4), 492–497.

20. Rieger, G., Linsenmeier, J. A., Gygax, L., & Bailey, J. M. (2008). Sexual orientation and childhood gender nonconformity: Evidence from home videos. *Developmental Psychology, 44*(1), 46–58.

Chapter 6

1. Masters, W. H., & Johnson, V. J. (1970). *Human sexual inadequacy.* Boston: Little, Brown and Company.

2. Sprecher, S., & Hendrick, S. S. (2004). Self-disclosure in intimate relationships: Associations with individual and relationship characteristics over time. *Journal of Social and Clinical Psychology, 23*(6), 857–877.

3. Laurenceau, J. P., Barrett, L. F., & Pietromonaco, P. R. (1998). Intimacy as an interpersonal process: The importance of self-disclosure, partner disclosure, and perceived partner responsiveness in interpersonal exchanges. *Journal of Personality and Social Psychology, 74*(5), 1238–1251.

4. Sprecher & Hendrick. Self-disclosure in intimate relationships.

5. Rehman, U. S., Rellini, A. H., & Fallis, E. (2011). The importance of sexual self-disclosure to sexual satisfaction and functioning in committed relationships. *Journal of Sexual Medicine, 8*(11), 3108–3115.

6. Birnbaum, G. E., Mizrahi, M., Kaplan, A., Kadosh, D., Kariv, D., Tabib, D., …& Burban, D. (2017). Sex unleashes your tongue: Sexual riming motivates self-disclosure to a new acquaintance and interest in future interactions. *Personality and Social Psychology Bulletin, 43*(5), 706–715.

7. Laurenceau, Barrett & Pietromonaco. Intimacy as an interpersonal process.

8. Greene, K., Derlega, V. J., & Mathews, A. (2006). Self-disclosure in personal relationships. In A. L. Vangelisti & D. Perlman (Eds.), *The Cambridge handbook of personal relationships* (pp. 409–427). New York: Cambridge University Press.

9. Birnbaum, Mizrahi, Kaplan, Kadosh, Kariv, Tabib,... & Burban. Sex unleashes your tongue.

10. Greene, Derlega, & Mathews. Self-disclosure in personal relationships.

11. Laurenceau, Barrett & Pietromonaco. Intimacy as an interpersonal process.

12. Aron, A., Melinat, E., Aron, E. N., Vallone, R. D., & Bator, R. J. (1997). The experimental generation of interpersonal closeness: A procedure and some preliminary findings. *Personality and Social Psychology Bulletin, 23*(4), 363–377.

Chapter 7

1. Steadman, H. J., Mulvey, E. P., Monahan, J., Robbins, P. C., Appelbaum, P. S., Grisso, T.,... Silver, E. (1998). Violence by people discharged from acute psychiatric inpatient facilities and by others in the same neighborhoods. *Archives of General Psychiatry, 55*, 393–401.

2. Although most people are aware of women's ability to have multiple orgasms, at least some men are capable of them, too. As recounted in a 1998 paper published in the *Journal of Sex Education and Therapy*, a thirty-five-year-old father of four gave a firsthand demonstration of this ability to a team of scientists by orgasming and ejaculating six times in thirty-six minutes as he sat in a laboratory watching porn.

   Whipple, B., Myers, B. R., & Komisaruk, B. R. (1998). Male multiple ejaculatory orgasms: A case study. *Journal of Sex Education and Therapy, 23*(2), 157–162.

3. Frederick, D. A., Lever, J., Gillespie, B. J., & Garcia, J. R. (2017). What keeps passion alive? Sexual satisfaction is associated with sexual communication, mood setting, sexual variety, oral sex, orgasm, and sex frequency in a national US study. *Journal of Sex Research, 54*(2), 186–201.

4. Monteiro Pascoal, P., Cardoso, D., & Henriques, R. (2015). Sexual satisfaction and distress in sexual functioning in a sample of the BDSM community: A comparison study between BDSM and non-BDSM contexts. *Journal of Sexual Medicine, 12*(4), 1052–1061.

5. Frappier, J., Toupin, I., Levy, J. J., Aubertin-Leheudre, M., & Karelis, A. D. (2013). Energy expenditure during sexual activity in young healthy couples. *PLOS ONE, 8*(10), e79342.

6. Haake, P., Krueger, T. H., Goebel, M. U., Heberling, K. M., Hartmann, U., & Schedlowski, M. (2004). Effects of sexual arousal on lymphocyte subset circulation and cytokine production in man. *Neuroimmunomodulation, 11*, 293–298.

7. Davey Smith, G., Frankel, S., & Yarnell, J. (1997). Sex and death: Are they related? Findings from the Caerphilly Cohort Study. *British Medical Journal, 315*, 1641–1644.

8. Maunder, L., Schoemaker, D., & Pruessner, J. C. (2016). Frequency of penile-vaginal intercourse is associated with verbal recognition performance in adult women. *Archives of Sexual Behavior, 46*, 441–453.

9. Wilson, T. D., & Gilbert, D. T. (2003). Affective forecasting. *Advances in Experimental Social Psychology, 35*, 345–411.

10. Miller, R. S. (1997). Inattentive and contented: Relationship commitment and attention to alternatives. *Journal of Personality and Social Psychology, 73*(4), 758–766.

11. Sagarin, B. J., Cutler, B., Cutler, N., Lawler-Sagarin, K. A., & Matuszewich, L. (2009). Hormonal changes and couple bonding in consensual sadomasochistic activity. *Archives of Sexual Behavior, 38*(2), 186–200.

12. Among the documented cases of BDSM-related deaths are an Ohio man who choked on a sex toy while he was bound and gagged and a Pennsylvania woman who was electrocuted by her husband while using electric nipple clamps.

    Lehmiller, J. (2013, October 7). Death by sex: Five of the most unusual sex-related deaths [Blog post]. Retrieved from https://www.lehmiller.com/blog/2013/10/7/death-by-sex-5-of-the-most-unusual-sex-related-deaths

13. Doctor, R., & Prince, V. (1997). Transvestism: A survey of 1,032 crossdressers. *Archives of Sexual Behavior, 26*, 589–605.

14. Prause, N., Steele, V. R., Staley, C., Sabatinelli, D., & Hajcak, G. (2015). Modulation of late positive potentials by sexual images in problem users and controls inconsistent with "porn addiction." *Biological Psychology, 109*, 192–199.

15. Sagarin, Cutler, Cutler, Lawler-Sagarin, & Matuszewich. Hormonal changes and couple bonding in consensual sadomasochistic activity.

16. Schmiedeberg, C., & Schröder, J. (2016). Does sexual satisfaction change with relationship duration? *Archives of Sexual Behavior, 45*, 99–107.

Chapter 8

1. Though marital happiness has declined for both men and women since the 1970s, the drop has been steeper for women. The number of men who described their marriage as "very happy" was 69.3 percent in 1974 and 62.8 percent in 2014. For women, the numbers were 68.4 percent and 57.4 percent, respectively.

   Smith, T. W., Son, J., & Schapiro, B. (2015, April). General social survey final report: Trends in psychological well-being. Retrieved from http://www.norc.org/PDFs/GSS%20Reports/GSS_PsyWellBeing15 _final_formatted.pdf

2. Schonfeld, Z. (2013, July 2). Wives are cheating 40% more than they used to, but still 70% as much as men. *The Atlantic*. Retrieved from https://www.theatlantic.com/national/archive/2013/07/wives-cheating -vs-men/313704/

3. Smith, Son, & Schapiro. General social survey final report: Trends in psychological well-being.

4. Amato, P. R., & Previti, D. (2003). People's reasons for divorcing: Gender, social class, the life course, and adjustment. *Journal of Family Issues, 24*(5), 602–626.

5. Kantor, L., & Levitz, N. (2017). Parents' views on sex education in schools: How much do Democrats and Republicans agree? *PLOS ONE, 12*(7), e0180250.

6. Allen, M., Emmers, T., Gebhardt, L., & Giery, M. A. (1995). Exposure to pornography and acceptance of rape myths. *Journal of Communication, 45*(1), 5–26; Tylka, T. L. (2015). No harm in looking, right?

Men's pornography consumption, body image, and well-being. *Psychology of Men & Masculinity, 16*(1), 97–107.

7. Frederick, D. A., Lever, J., Gillespie, B. J., & Garcia, J. R. (2017). What keeps passion alive? Sexual satisfaction is associated with sexual communication, mood setting, sexual variety, oral sex, orgasm, and sex frequency in a national US study. *Journal of Sex Research, 54*(2), 186–201.

8. Alford, S., & Hauser, D. (2011). *Adolescent sexual health in Europe and the US* (4th ed.). Advocates for Youth. Retrieved from http://www.advocatesforyouth.org/component/content/article/419-adolescent-sexual-health-in-europe-and-the-us

9. Weaver, H., Smith, G., & Kippax, S. (2005). School-based sex education policies and indicators of sexual health among young people: A comparison of the Netherlands, France, Australia and the United States. *Sex Education, 5*, 171–188.

10. In the 2017 World Happiness Report, the Netherlands was ranked sixth and the United States fourteenth out of fifteen countries.

    Gilchrist, K. (2017, March 20). These are the 15 happiest countries in the world. *CNBC*. Retrieved from https://www.cnbc.com/2017/03/20/norway-ranked-worlds-happiest-country-as-the-us-gets-sadder.html

11. "No promo homo" laws. (n.d.) GLSEN. Retrieved from https://www.glsen.org/learn/policy/issues/nopromohomo

12. Weaver, Smith, & Kippax. School-based sex education policies and indicators of sexual health among young people.

13. Stanger-Hall, K. F., & Hall, D. W. (2011). Abstinence-only education and teen pregnancy rates: Why we need comprehensive sex education in the US. *PLOS ONE, 6*(10), e24658.

14. Veale, D., Miles, S., Bramley, S., Muir, G., & Hodsoll, J. (2015). Am I normal? A systematic review and construction of nomograms for flaccid and erect penis length and circumference in up to 15,521 men. *BJU International, 115*(6), 978–986.

15. Gailliot, M. T., & Baumeister, R. F. (2007). Self-regulation and sexual restraint: Dispositionally and temporarily poor self-regulatory

abilities contribute to failures at restraining sexual behavior. *Personality and Social Psychology Bulletin, 33*(2), 173–186.

16. Berlin, F. S., Maim, H. M., & Dean, S. (1991). Effects of statutes requiring psychiatrists to report. *American Journal of Psychiatry, 148*(4), 449–453.

17. A Marist poll conducted around Valentine's Day, 2011, found that 73 percent of Americans believed in the concept of a soulmate, up from 66 percent the previous summer. Persons under thirty had the highest rate of belief in a soulmate (80 percent).

    "It's destiny!" Most Americans believe in soul mates. (2011, February 10). *Marist Poll.* Retrieved from http://maristpoll.marist. edu/210-its-destiny-most-americans-believe-in-soul-mates/

18. Dew, J. (2009). Has the marital time cost of parenting changed over time? *Social Forces, 88,* 519–541.

19. Knee, C. R. (1998). Implicit theories of relationships: Assessment and prediction of romantic relationship initiation, coping, and longevity. *Journal of Personality and Social Psychology, 74*(2), 360–370.

20. Le, B., Dove, N. L., Agnew, C. R., Korn, M. S., & Mutso, A. A. (2010). Predicting nonmarital romantic relationship dissolution: A meta-analytic synthesis. *Personal Relationships, 17*(3), 377–390.

21. Passion typically declines between six and thirty months after the start of a relationship, though it is possible to keep passion alive beyond this time period by continually introducing novelty into the relationship.

    Hatfield, E., & Walster, W. G. (1978). *A new look at love.* Lanham, MD: University Press of America.

22. Meston, C. M., & Frohlich, P. F. (2003). Love at first fright: Partner salience moderates roller-coaster-induced excitation transfer. *Archives of Sexual Behavior, 32*(6), 537–544.

23. Rubel, A. N., & Bogaert, A. F. (2015). Consensual nonmonogamy: Psychological well-being and relationship quality correlates. *Journal of Sex Research, 52*(9), 961–982.

24. Balzarini, R. N., Campbell, L., Kohut, T., Holmes, B. M., Lehmiller, J. J., Harman, J. J., & Atkins, N. (2017). Perceptions of primary and secondary relationships in polyamory. *PLOS ONE, 12*(5), e0177841.

Index